THE SPOT REDUCING DIET

THE SPOT REDUCING DIET

A Beverly Hills Nutritionist
Tells You How To Lose Weight
Where You Want To

Hermien Lee with Linda Lane

Coward-McCann, Inc.
New York

Copyright © 1983 by Hermien Lee and Linda Lane
All rights reserved. This book, or parts thereof, may not be reproduced in any form without permission in writing from the publisher. Published on the same day in Canada by General Publishing Co. Limited, Toronto.

Library of Congress Cataloging in Publication Data

Lee, Hermien.
The spot reducing diet.

1. Reducing diets. I. Lane, Linda. II. Title.
RM222.2.L415   1983   613.2'5   83-14264
ISBN 0-698-11243-1

Printed in the United States of America

Fourth Impression

ACKNOWLEDGMENTS

It has taken many years and thousands of clients to prove that losing weight where you want to—spot reducing—is possible. It is my wonderful clients who triggered the connection between *what* one eats and *where* it affects the body.

Writing a book takes enormous intestinal fortitude, lots of support from friends and family, the patience of Job, and a workaholic's unconditional love and devotion. It takes cooperation on all levels. When we began the Spot Reducing Diet, Robin Beard very generously edited our presentation. Tom Miller recognized the potential of spot reducing and became our editor at Coward-McCann.

I would like to thank everyone who was kind enough to be interviewed during the course of writing and compiling the information for the book. Many of you are mentioned by name and I appreciate your willingness to help people understand that you can control your shape as well as your weight. I would also like to thank those of you who were interested but either chose not to be named or had to be left out because of editorial space-saving decisions. It is you, my clients, who have made my revolutionary theories a wonderful reality and I thank you.

My children got me out of the kitchen and back into the work force. Then Ron Fletcher believed in me and gave me my start in private practice as a Beverly Hills nutritionist. I will always be grateful to Ron for expanding my life and my horizons. I would like to thank my friend, nutrition expert Dr. Judith Ashley, for reading the manuscript with an eye for accuracy.

The recipes have been tested and retested, and if you think too many cooks can spoil the broth, this is one instance in which two of them—Jill Boris and Jennifer Gilbert—have greatly enhanced it.

A special thanks to Katharine Ross for helping us when we needed it most. To Nancy Andrews for being a terrific photographer. To Lee Ann Chearneyi for putting the finishing editorial touches on the manuscript, and revving us up to go on the road. And thanks to screenwriter Ivan Moffat for his enthusiasm and pointers on playing chess with food.

Special thanks to Barbara ("Missy") Huger for her patience, perseverance, and expertise as a production supervisor; and to Millie Loeb for her support and advice.

And especially, I would like to thank screenwriter Linda Lane, without whom the information in this book would have reached only my individual clients. After going through the program, Linda had the vision and confidence to compile, write, and produce my theories into *The Spot Reducing Diet*.

H.L.

TO OUR CHILDREN:

Dwight Eisenhower Lee
Dr. John Hughes Lee
Dr. William Myers Lee
Jane Lee Weiland

Lucy Lane Harrison

CONTENTS

INTRODUCTION   11

The Basics   17

1 • Hit the Spot   19
2 • How to Be a Successful Dieter   32

THE MASTER PLAN   43

3 • The Spot Reducing Master Plan Program   45
4 • A Spot Reducing Month of Menus   58

HIT THE SPOT!   83

5 • The Face and Neck   85
6 • Shoulders   94
7 • Arms   98
8 • Breasts   101
9 • The Back   105
10 • The Stomach and Waistline   108
11 • Posterior, Hips, Thighs, Saddlebags, and Calves   117
12 • Face to Feet   124
13 • The Biggest Offenders for Each Body Spot   128

HIT THE SPOT RECIPES   133

14 • Low-Calorie Gourmet Dishes   135

THE SPOT REDUCING DIET AS A WAY OF LIFE   165

15 • Dining Out   167
16 • Travel   182
17 • Pregnancy   189
18 • Nursing   198
19 • Overweight Children and Teenagers   205

EXERCISES   215

20 • Ron Fletcher's Exercise Guide   217

MAINTENANCE   221

21 • Maintenance   223

APPENDIX A

Questions and Answers   229

APPENDIX B

About Your Body   234

INTRODUCTION

Twenty years ago I weighed 170 pounds and wore a size 20 dress. I was a middle-aged housewife with training in nutrition, four children, and a history of going up and down the scale like a yoyo. I looked like a bloated rag doll—overstuffed above and below the waist and tightly tied in the middle. I was so out of touch with my body that I didn't know how overweight and out-of-proportion I was until I caught a glimpse of myself in a store window. I wondered who this big, fat horse was. . . . I turned around and much to my surprise, I was the only one standing there. I was horrified!

Why would anyone want to pay a fat nutritionist to tell her how to lose weight? Visions of an empty waiting room meshed with visions of an empty appointment book, and I knew it was time for me to lose weight once and for all.

I devised the Spot Reducing Diet, went on it, and over a period of months I slimmed down 60 pounds. When I reached my goal weight of 110 pounds I was a beautifully proportioned size 4. All the ugly lumps, bumps, and bulges—*spots*, as I call them—had disappeared along with my bad eating habits. I felt years younger and, had I not spent years going from deprivation to reward—starving myself and then bingeing—I would have looked ten years younger as well.

The best way to prevent sagging, bagging, and wrinkling is to lose weight *slowly*, eat a nutritious balance of protein, fat, and carbohydrate, and then maintain your goal weight and shape on a permanent basis.

If you are older and it's too late for preventive measures, you will be encouraged to know that my skin is tighter and more youthful today than it was 20 years ago. Following my Maintenance Program, I have become more emotionally centered—no more high/low mood swings—and I have been able to maintain my goal weight and spot-free shape.

An exciting difference between the Spot Reducing Diet and other diets is that now, for the first time, you will be able to turn to the chapter on the part or parts of your body that you want to reduce or reshape. Whether it's two pounds' worth of saddlebags or 200 pounds of excess fat from head to foot, a paunchy stomach, fat arms, or a puffy face, you will learn what caused your problem and how to correct it.

Your body is the most wonderful computer in the world; when you treat it well you will achieve a symbiotic relationship between body and mind. You will discover new tastes and textures. Quality will become more important than quantity. And once you have achieved your goal weight and shape, you will learn how to maintain them forever by making the Maintenance Program part of your life. Maintenance means being able to eat or drink anything you can control.

Many of my clients are models, actors, and actresses whose livelihood depends on a naturally radiant appearance and a high level of energy. As they discovered, the Spot Reducing Diet is not just a diet, it is a wonderful way of life. I know that I would not be as effective at what I do today had I not overcome a history of being overweight and out of proportion myself.

When I was a child growing up in Illinois my mother was a member of the local Cream and Butter Brigade. That meant that only the thickest creamery butter was used in our home and when my mother made one pie, she made eight. My sister Julie and I were a couple of sugar addicts and butterballs; no matter how hard we tried, no matter how many diets were started and even followed, we always ended up going back to our old eating habits and our old shapes. In early photographs I bear a strong resemblance to Sitting Bull.

It wasn't until I went off to the University of Illinois to study chemistry and nutrition that I lost weight. I was just too busy to eat between meals. The excess weight melted away and by the time I received my Bachelor of Science degree I was thin.

The miracle didn't last for long. I took my internship in dietetics at Michael Reese Hospital in Chicago. One of our responsibilities was to close the kitchen at night. We were allowed to eat what we wanted before storing the leftovers. Well, amazing as this seems, we had a wonderful French chef who created dishes for the exclusive private unit. By the time we had our fill of veal Oscar and cherries jubilee there were no leftovers. The closer we came to getting our degrees the bigger our class became—and I don't mean in numbers.

By the time I went off to Johns Hopkins in Baltimore I was a well-educated butterball. I spent two years as a ward dietitian before joining their hospital unit and spending the next three and half years working in Australia, New Guinea, and the Dutch East Indies.

During World War II, I was a very young, very plump lieutenant in the Medical Corps stationed in Sydney, Australia, as a supervising dietitian. While I was waiting for our hospital to be completed, I spent a lot of time overeating Devonshire cream tea—hot baking powder biscuits stuffed with strawberry jam and swimming in heavy cream. Contrary to all my knowledge as a dietitian, I had allowed my craving for sugar to rule my life. My sugar addiction was in full swing. I was 5'3" tall and I weighed 165 pounds.

"Hermien," a friend said, "I've got just the man for you!"

"Wait!" I insisted. "I can't meet anybody until I lose weight!"

"Oh, yes, you can. This is someone special. He's Colonel Tex Lee, Eisenhower's senior aide. You'll have to meet him through the mail first—you'll have plenty of time to go on a diet!"

Our correspondence began. Tex and I became very close in the accelerated fashion that so often took place during the war. We shared our hopes, dreams, fears, and, of course, our photographs. Naturally, I found an old, slim, pre-Devonshire cream tea photo to send. I kept swearing to myself that I would begin my diet *tomorrow*.

The war was winding down and I was being sent back to the States. I informed Colonel Lee and he wrote back proposing marriage. If we felt the same when we met as we did when we communicated through the mail he wanted to marry me immediately. He would meet me in Chicago in six weeks. Six weeks! I had a little over one month to lose 50 pounds.

During the cruise home I starved myself and when we reached Chicago I looked like the slim girl in the photograph. It was a much too rapid weight loss, but love knows no bounds and as it turned out, Colonel Tex Lee was the love of my life. We were married one week after meeting.

Tex and I moved to Indianapolis and had four children. My family became my life. Then, as the children grew up, I decided it was time to resume my career as a nutritionist.

Our home served as my office and, at first, my clients were friends and neighbors. Word-of-mouth spread throughout our community; within two years I saw 500 people. It was during this period that I discovered spot reducing.

In the '50s we did diets according to the weight of food. No one ever dreamed that the shape of his or her body was a direct result of what they ate. If anything, your shape was thought to be hereditary. Genetics were blamed for big billboard behinds, padded-looking shoulders, thick calves, a double chin, or a straight up and down, no-waistline shape.

What triggered my spot-reducing concept was that clients who had always had a big behind or a big stomach were able to lose weight in those specific spots by changing their eating habits, *by balancing their nutrients*. Since we tend to eat the same way our parents ate it stood to reason that people who came from families who were overweight and out of proportion, now had the ability to break their unattractive molds.

For several years I kept records of my clients' measurements as well as their weights. I discovered that in case after case consuming too much carbohydrate caused people to get a paunchy stomach, a big diaphragm, fat arms, a puffy face, and backfuls of flesh. The lovers of fat, the people who ate their food fried and their beef with lots of marbling, drank gallons of milk shakes, and couldn't resist butter or mayonnaise had big hips and thighs, even fat knees. The protein overeaters, the people who ate big, hearty slabs of beef, cartons of cottage cheese and yogurt, and cheese, found themselves big and seemingly muscular all over. It also seemed that a combination of fat and carbohydrate, things like ice cream, potato chips, and buttery cake, were what caused the dimpled fat often referred to as *cellulite*.

To prove that we are what we eat, I restructured my clients' diets. If they ate a properly balanced diet their bodies would eliminate the out-of-proportion spot or spots. *A balanced diet produced a balanced shape*.

Spot reducing, losing weight *only* where you want to, seemed like a wild and revolutionary idea. I wasn't sure why this form of body sculpture worked, but I watched the same patterns and results occurring with each successive client. It also became clear that big sugar eaters like myself were sugar addicts. And big fat eaters, many of whom had no idea how much fat and oil they consumed because much of it was hidden or invisible to begin with, were fat addicts. Rebalancing their diets meant experiencing a form of withdrawal no less dramatic than nicotine withdrawal.

My two years of working with clients at home as well as losing 60 pounds myself prepared me to go back to work. I began as an assistant pediatric dietitian dealing with extreme cases of overweight and underweight individuals in Riley Hospital at Indiana University Medical Center. In 1971 I moved to California to join a research team at Martin Luther King, Jr. Hospital in Los Angeles.

Just before visiting Indiana in 1975, quite by chance I visited Ron Fletcher's Beverly Hills exercise studio. Ron Fletcher was famous for shaping, toning, and in some cases reshaping some of Hollywood's biggest film and television stars. Candace Bergen, Ali McGraw, Katharine Ross, and Ben Vereen are a few of the stars featured on the cover of Ron's exercise book, *Every Body Is Beautiful*.

We discussed my revolutionary approach to spot reducing and diet. Ron liked it and explained that there were times when an actor, actress, or model would arrive on his doorstep with a body so totally out of shape in one spot or another that although there might be three or four weeks before the cameras started rolling, there was a limit to what he could change with exercise in such a short time. He suggested that we combine forces. "If you can reshape the body through diet," he told me, "in some cases you'll be performing a miracle!"

That day in 1975 proved to be a turning point in my life. I opened an office adjacent to Ron's exercise studio. Teaching people how to look and feel their best became my business. My first client was television and stage star Sandy Duncan. She wanted to smooth her upper, outer thighs. Saddlebags, no matter how unobtrusive, are still noticeable on film. Sandy learned to hit her spot and she's been streamlined ever since.

To date I have worked with some 4000 clients ranging in age from eight to eighty-three. Children and adults of all ages and from every social and economic background have proven that there is a direct correlation between what you eat and where it goes on the body.

Losing weight is easy. It's losing it where you want and keeping it off permanently that sets the Spot Reducing Diet apart from other programs. The reason my clients pay $450 for 14 sessions is that they know that if they follow the principles outlined in this book, principles based on over 40 years of academic and professional experience, they will be able to maintain their good looks, good health, and good habits *forever*. Spot reducing is a revolutionary approach to body sculpture that is also safe, sensible, and delicious.

THE BASICS

1
HIT THE SPOT

The human body is the most amazing instrument I know of. When it is properly nourished with a balance of protein, fat, and carbohydrate it functions smoothly. When it is forced to adjust to an imbalance of one or more of those nutrients it develops bumps and bulges—*spots*.

Reducing or eliminating those spots means rebalancing your nutrients. By referring to the chapter or chapters that correspond to the spots you want to trim you will discover what caused your imbalance, how to correct it, and how to avoid getting it back in the future.

What Causes Your Spots

Fifty calories per meal more than your body needs, or 150 extra calories a day, will cause you to gain 15 pounds in one year. If you overeat carbohydrate you can have spots from the stomach up: a bulging midriff, a thick waistline, a big diaphragm, a fat back, big arms, a round face, and a thick neck. If you overeat protein you may be big and seemingly muscular all over, although I have some clients who have an overstuffed look only in the shoulders as a result of eating too much protein. Too much fat will give a person big spots from the waist down: a huge behind, big hips and thighs, saddlebags, thick calves, and fat knees.

Saddlebags are a particularly unattractive variation on the fat theme. They are caused by foods high in hidden as well as obvious fat. Things like chocolate mousse, butter cookies, and potato chips.

Actress Jean Kasem was amazed to see the dramatic difference in her legs after being on the program only a short time. She explains, "Every time I went on a fad diet—and I tried them all—I always lost weight from the waist up, and that's not where women want to lose. I went on the Spot Reducing Diet and within a week there was a noticeable change in my hips and thighs alone."

Bingeing

Bingeing is eating or drinking out of control: taking one bite and not being able to stop until you've finished the whole thing; opening a bottle of wine to have a glass and drinking the whole bottle. Bingeing is one of the major reasons the body gets out of proportion. When we overindulge we tend to do it with foods and beverages that fall into the same group. The lover of fat may think he can eat six peanuts, but once he's opened the can or dipped into a dish of them there's no stopping him until they're all gone.

The body handles a little much better than it handles a lot. It's far better to eat two small cookies every day, bad though cookies are for your shape, than 14 small cookies in one day. A lot causes big spots. And quickly! A little will add up to spots over a period of time.

Deprivation to Reward—Yoyoing

Losing a few pounds and then gaining them back, repeatedly going from deprivation to reward, is one way that people get a pear shape. Being small on top and big on the bottom can occur early in life, so many people believe that they are destined to be bottom-heavy and out of proportion forever. It's not true.

It doesn't matter if you are young, middle-aged, or old enough to have sagging, wrinkled skin from starving and then rewarding yourself—once you break this yoyoing pattern you will be able to lose weight evenly, to achieve a beautifully proportioned body even if you've never had one in your life. And your skin will tighten up.

Two Shapes at the Same Weight

If you take two people who are the same age, sex, height, bone structure, and weight, but one of them has a history of yoyoing and overindulging in protein, fat, or carbohydrate, while the other eats a well balanced diet and is careful to lose weight slowly when the occasion arises, you will see two people with two very different shapes. One will be well proportioned, while the other one may be bottom-heavy and will have one or more out-of-proportion spots.

Losing weight and losing weight where you want are usually two different exercises. I want you to think of your weight and your shape as being of equal importance. Don't make the scale your god. Lose weight *slowly* if you are going to lose it evenly. If you reach your goal weight before you achieve your perfect shape, be patient. Keep going and stick with the program until you have achieved both goals.

Changing Your Spots

To prove that you are what you eat, I think you should meet Gwyn. She was a real Mrs. Saddlebags, a forty-year-old woman who arrived in my office wearing a muumuu and shaped like a bell. Most of her weight was from the waist down.

Gwyn was bottom-heavy because she ate too much fat and oil. She loved fried chicken, chips and guacamole, and lots of cheese, by itself or on top of other food. "You're addicted to fat and oil," I told her. She was shocked. "I didn't know you could be addicted to fat. I thought you could only be addicted to sugar."

Over the next three months Gwyn hit her spots and ate a balanced diet. She began by weighing her protein and measuring her fat and carbohydrate so that she would eventually be able to look at a plate of food and know approximately how much of each she was getting. The muumuus were replaced by jeans. When Gwyn left my office she was a perfectly proportioned size 12.

One year later, Gwyn arrived at my office wearing another muumuu. She turned sideways and looked at me with tears in her eyes. "Are you pregnant?" I asked. "No," she said shaking her head. "I stopped eating fat. I became a vegetarian—and look at me. Vegetables aren't supposed to be fattening."

Vegetables eaten in moderation are not fattening. They're one of the best sources of vitamins and minerals. But like anything else, too much of anything good can be bad. Gwyn had become a carbohydrate overeater. She was eating far too much fruit, far too many vegetables and whole grains. She went back on the program and in a few weeks the only spare tire she had was in the trunk of her car.

The Right Balance

I emphasize eating the right balance of nutrients. That means always having meals with protein, fat and carbohydrate, vitamins and minerals.

When you eat a carbohydrate without a protein, your energy rises quickly, then falls abruptly. The reason you should include protein or fat is that they break down more slowly. They give you continued energy and staying power. When you eat a well-balanced diet you don't have to think about artificial energizers or junk food, which are better fuel for television commercials than for your body.

As you may have guessed, it's knowing which foods fall into the three categories that is going to give you the ability to make the right choices for yourself. Every body is unique. Every body responds differently to food and drink. Tune in to your body. Listen to what it's telling you and you'll know which foods to stay away from and which ones to eat often. And remember: never eat a carbohydrate without a protein unless you're going to bed, in which case the exhaustion after the sugar rush will help you sleep.

Variety

There are at least 55 nutrients that you need daily and the very best way to get them every day is by eating a variety of food. I want you to eat a little of a lot, not a lot of a little. I want you to have variety and to learn that food does not have to be rich to taste good. In the carbohydrate and protein categories there are many foods that are low in calories and still provide great taste and texture.

Many of these foods contain more than one element. A food rich in carbohydrate might contain protein as well. I don't want to confuse you with lengthy scientific explanations, but if you eat the same things every day you're not going to get a wide enough range.

The more creative you are when planning your meals the more successful you will be at dieting, and the more nutrients you will be ingesting. Besides, eating the same foods only leads to boredom. Take a good look at the Exchange Lists (p. 52) to appreciate the full extent to which you can be creative.

Eating a variety of vegetables, both fresh and frozen, seasonal and not, will allow you to expand your culinary horizon. Be daring, try new tastes and textures. I guarantee, whether or not you like vegetables and fruit now, by the time you have achieved your beautifully balanced body you will. Most of my clients begin the program by barely tolerating many of the things I insist they eat. After a few weeks most of them are amazed at just how many delicious foods they've spent years ignoring.

Moderation

Moderation is defined as restraint, keeping within proper limits, avoiding extremes; as in a moderate drinker, a moderate repast. It's easy for the dictionary to tell us what is moderate, but it's difficult for most of us to decide where to draw the line between moderate and excessive.

Alan Hamel came to me ten years ago. He wanted to lose 25 pounds *evenly* and without suffering the I'm-on-a-diet-too-thin-face syndrome. Moderation had no meaning for him. "My problem was I just never stopped eating. Food was never farther away than the length of my arm. The moment I went to watch television I ate something. It was automatic. I always carried food in the car and I could never drive past a fruit stand without stopping. My night table was a little minimarket. But until I went to Hermien I wasn't aware that my eating habits were excessive."

Telling the public where to buy their groceries and being married to television star Suzanne Somers, who just happens to be a gourmet cook, made it impossible for Alan to lose where he wanted. The first thing he had to do was learn the true meaning of moderation and change his eating habits accordingly. "I stopped eating between meals," Alan says. "For the first four or five years I ate three meals a day. Always sitting at the table. I started to have a real awareness of how my body interacted with food. Now, ten years later, I've stopped using salt, sugar, creamery products, chocolate, and salad dressing. I've come to appreciate the taste of vegetables. Suzanne and I have both eliminated the foods that affected us adversely."

Alan reached his goal weight and shape years ago. "The Spot Reducing Diet really changed my life because it showed me a way around bad times other than with food. I feel better now than I did ten years ago."

Your Appestat

According to Dorland's Illustrated Medical Dictionary your *appestat* is "A center in the hypothalmus that reacts to a shortage of calories by promoting hunger and causing a desire for food, and reacts to food intake by inducing a feeling of satiety."

Your appestat acts like a thermostat. When your thermostat is broken you find yourself in one uncomfortable room after another. When your appestat is out of whack you receive a continuous message: "Feed me—feed me—feed me!"

When your appestat is working properly, it signals you when it is time to eat. "Feed me!," grumbles your stomach. "I'm feeling weak, I think I should eat something." "The lunch bell—I'm starving!" You get the message and you eat. It takes approximately 20 minutes for your appestat to get the message that you are full. If you gobble your food, the chances are that you will eat more than you need. Eating more slowly will help to keep your appestat in good working order.

My biggest challenge was Joy. Joy was 5'3" tall and—after a trip to the stockyards because my doctor's scale wouldn't go high enough—we calculated her weight at 400 pounds. She was a cheerful woman married to a prominent dentist and they had two thin, healthy children.

Joy could eat a whole turkey with stuffing at one sitting. And when she traveled around the country giving speeches on adoption she wanted to be fair to every fast-food operation. She would begin with the first restaurant, a Bob's Big Boy or a Burger King, and work her way down the main drag, stopping at each and every establishment. She would have a Foster's Freeze and French fries. Her appestat was so out of whack that she was never full.

It took two years to trim nearly 200 pounds off Joy and get her appestat communicating once again. Knowing when you have had enough is one of the major keys to losing weight and keeping it off.

Sugar, the Big Reward

Americans eat an average of 109 pounds of sugar per person each year. How sweet it is—your coffee, your sugar-frosted flakes, and ice cream. We have been raised on sugar, and we still think of it as the quintessential reward. When you were good you were rewarded with candy, cake, and ice cream. When you were bad you couldn't have dessert. Early on, the power of sugar and its immediate gratification and reward values were established. Take away the sugar and you take away the prize. Take away the alcohol and you remove your right to relax. There are so many ways to rationalize consuming too many carbohydrates.

The first bite you take is psychological. You want a taste of something sweet, birthday cake, a cookie, a sip of wine. Then, because of insulin, the second bite becomes physiological. Insulin is sugar-hungry. The islets of Langerhans, which are located in the pancreas, are little glands that manufacture insulin. The insulin has to balance the sugar. This creates a seesaw effect: your blood sugar rises, you have a burst of energy, then your energy wanes, and you need more, so you want another glass of beer or wine or another handful of pretzels. You're suddenly tired again so you consume more carbohydrates and the self-perpetuating cycle continues. You may not even realize that you're a sugar addict.

There are good carbohydrates and bad carbohydrates. Fruits, vegetables, and whole grains are good because they carry vitamins and minerals as well as sugar. But the sugar in fruit can be the same as candy, definitely a bad, empty carbohydrate, if you eat too much of it. Too much of anything means spots.

When you put food in your mouth, make sure it's something that supplies vitamins and minerals. Think with your brain, not with your taste buds.

Sugar Withdrawal

Do you suffer from severe mood swings—one minute you're elated and the next you're down in the dumps and you don't know why? Do you snap at your children for no good reason? Do you tire easily?

The chances are you are suffering from *sugar withdrawal*, the curse of the sugar addict.

Suzanne Somers, who used to be a sugar and a fat addict, told me, "I think more clearly and my moods are more balanced when I follow the program. If I have sugar now I get mood swings. The other day I was having a sugar fit and my son had some Reese's peanut butter cups, which he had been selling on the beach. I decided to have one—well, it's peanut butter and not much chocolate. . . . The next day I was agitated and I found myself snapping a couple of times. I know that little bit of sugar made me nervous."

I have so many clients, including doctors, who have never made the correlation between giving up sugar—and I don't mean the sugar in fruits and vegetables—and being physically and emotionally overwhelmed for a period of weeks. Dr. Lesley Z. Blumberg, a Beverly Hills gynecologist, came to me to trim her saddlebags and to learn how to maintain her perfectly balanced figure once she had hit her spot. Lesley went on the program and she stopped eating foods with added sugar. All too quickly she experienced *sugar withdrawal*.

Lesley explained, "I have had the experience of eating a high-sugar meal at breakfast and feeling fine for about thirty minutes or an hour and suddenly starting to have the symptoms of jitters, a racing pulse, headache; all the things you would experience if you got too much insulin on board and really dropped your blood sugar. So, I'm convinced that it's an absolute necessity that if you're going to eat any carbohydrate at breakfast, or if you're going to eat a piece of fruit between meals, you should have an ounce of protein to balance it to keep your blood sugar up at all times."

This is one of the reasons I stress following the program *exactly*. The Spot Reducing Diet is a well balanced diet that will *help* you get through sugar withdrawal. You don't have to experience severe mood swings if you know how to counteract them.

Dr. Blumberg says, "Snacking in a way that will maintain your blood sugar—by dividing your protein portions throughout the day, including at snack time as well as meals—you can avoid getting highs and lows. That means that by balancing your nutrients you will be more balanced emotionally."

Sugar, in its wide variety of forms, can seem like your very best friend. Mary isn't always there, Bob isn't always there, but sugar is.

Sugar is as near or as far as you put it. And when you put it out of reach, your body may go into a mourning state.

To counteract sugar withdrawal, combine a carbohydrate with a protein—a carrot with a teaspoon of specially prepared peanut butter (see p. 79) or an apple with a piece of partial skim milk cheese. A bite of foods in the right combination will give you a feeling of well-being, a second wind that will help you through quite stressful moments.

It takes about three weeks to get through the withdrawal symptoms. One of my clients, actress Julie Carmen, really suffered with sugar withdrawal. "It took me two months to really get over the craving for sugar, and it was intense. I went through a period for a week when I was feverish and sweaty. I had to burn the sugar out of my system. Now, when I feel deprived or blue or depressed about something, I think ahead and have a sugar substitute ready. When everybody else is having ice cream or cheesecake I can put a drop of milk in my coffee and feel that I'm giving myself a treat."

Once you've conquered your addiction, as with giving up cigarettes, you will feel so much more centered, calm, and charged with vitality that even when you're tempted you'll know how far you can go without becoming addicted all over again. *Moderation is the dividing line between you and your sugar or fat addiction.*

A mother brought her paunchy eight-year-old hyperactive son to me as a last resort. The boy was one of six and his brothers and sisters were all bright and easy to manage, but Robert was like a jack-in-the-box. He couldn't concentrate on any one thing for more than a minute. His teachers even suggested that he just wasn't bright and perhaps should be placed in a remedial class.

We analyzed the boy's eating habits and discovered that he was eating an average of eight pieces of fruit a day, handfuls of jelly beans, plus a couple of soft drinks. There were colorful jars of jelly beans in the kitchen and living room. There was a large basket of fresh fruit in the kitchen—a communal feast for a very large family— and the refrigerator was well stocked with soft drinks. No one calculated or watched to see who ate what, so Robert just ate and ate and ate until he had a terrible carbohydrate imbalance. He was overdosing on sugar. The boy agreed to limit his daily fruit consumption to two pieces. To help him help himself, his mother removed the jelly beans and soft drinks from the house.

Removing temptation is a big help, but motivation and reward are two more factors that play a role in changing your eating habits. In Robert's case we were able to enlist the aid of his teacher. She asked him to give his classmates a two-minute daily lecture on nutrition. Instead of the negative attention "the fat boy" was used to receiving, he began getting positive attention. He would call me to give me a progress report and to get more information for his classroom lectures.

After a few weeks Robert's fat stomach leveled off and his personality changed completely. He could concentrate on his lessons and could even sit still and read a book while his mother talked to me. He was no longer the dumb fat boy; he was bright, slim, and energetic. At the end of the school term his grades went from D's to A's.

You may say, "Hey, wait a minute! My favorite foods are carbohydrates." Fine, so are mine. When you know how to balance your diet you will be able to eat anything within moderation.

Some doctors say sugar or fat addiction is psychological; others treat it as a physical addiction on the order of alcohol or nicotine dependence. There are seven symptoms to the withdrawal syndrome: you may be suffering withdrawal if you frequently get very tired, very hungry, weak, shaky, irritable, depressed, or headachy.

Fat

When it comes to fat, you are what you eat. The typical American diet consists of 40 percent fat. It's tucked away where it can't be seen. Butter, margarine, salad oil, and highly fatted meats account for less than one half of the fat we consume.

Fat addiction is as bad and difficult to break as any other addiction. And sometimes it's worse, because people don't even know that they have it. Fat is insidious—it's used in so many dishes and is part of so many foods that we never think of as being particularly loaded with it. I have many clients who tell me, "I don't understand why you think I eat too much fat! I don't eat bacon, and I use only one teaspoon of diet margarine a day." Then we do a food history and we find out that they've been eating cheese, nuts, seeds, avocados, and that they drink low-fat, not nonfat, milk.

A classic example of this hidden fat comes up when you roast potatoes and carrots around a leg of lamb. They soak up the oil as they get crisp and brown. The fact that the potatoes seem dry doesn't mean that they're not loaded with oil. A croissant melts in your mouth because it's loaded with butter. When you order a breaded dish and remove the breading, you are still getting far too much oil that has soaked into the food.

Just as with sugar addiction, you'll discover that once you've kicked the habit you won't enjoy foods loaded with butter and oil.

The body is very thrifty. The liver produces enough bile, which is stored in the gall bladder, to accommodate your usual daily intake of fat. It is secreted as needed. If you suddenly throw a big load of oil into your system, it has to compensate by producing more bile.

What you've done to your body is as shocking as being awakened by a bucket of ice water in the morning. The result is that you will probably feel physically ill, sometimes for a few hours, sometimes for a few days.

Body Types—Endomorphic, Mesomorphic, Ectomorphic

Some of you may argue that you were born fat and there's nothing you can do about it, that you gain weight even when you only look inside a bakery, even when you're being moderate.

"If I look at a piece of cheesecake I gain weight." I've heard that one at least 400 times. In fact, I've heard every story, every variation on every fat theme, known to man. And after years of analyzing stories and people I've discovered that fat is not as hereditary as you think.

Fat cells start forming when the fetus is six months along. And if the mother-to-be stuffs herself with fattening junk food the child is going to be born with a correspondingly large number of fat cells. The more fat cells you have, the greater chance you have of being overweight.

Fat cells are like grape clusters. You can empty them but you can never get rid of them. Doctors believe that we continue to make fat cells until we're 20. This is another point for science to ponder. We don't know exactly how long we continue to manufacture them but we are 100 percent certain that it is these fat cells that make the difference between gaining weight easily or not.

The endomorph has a round body type that gains weight easily, with lots of fat cells waiting to be filled up. The mesomorph is more angular; although he has to watch his weight, he can afford to be more carefree than the endomorph. Ectomorphs are the ones to be envied. They appear to eat and drink whatever they please and they never seem to gain an ounce. Many gangling, leggy models are ectomorphs. Of course they do gain weight, but when they do it's usually very slowly.

By the time your body type has been determined—endomorphic, mesomorphic, or ectomorphic—you will have an idea how much overeating and overdrinking you can get away with.

We must realize that we have fat cells that can be emptied and can even seem to disappear altogether, but it's only an illusion. Those nasty empty fat cells are just waiting to be filled up again. When you lose weight they shrink, but they will always be a part of you. Even when you have reached your well proportioned goal you must consider yourself *reformed, but never cured.* You will always have to be aware of what caused you to gain weight in a specific area and which foods and beverages you must continuously monitor to prevent another imbalance.

Your Biggest Reward

Even at the best of times, regimenting your intake of food and drink makes people sigh, "Oh, no—I don't want to . . . but I guess I should." It doesn't seem particularly rewarding at the start. That's why quick-weight-loss diets are so popular. People want an overnight miracle, but the truth is that you can't expect lasting results unless you're willing to change your eating habits.

Bobby Colomby, formerly the drummer with the rock group Blood, Sweat and Tears, came to me to lose weight all over. When he was ready for maintenance, 50 pounds later, he reflected on the program. "The rewards were automatic. You give off a very powerful, positive energy that people want to be part of. Why does anyone become overweight? It's because he's lost his self-esteem. Forget habit. It's self-esteem, because if you had it you wouldn't *have* the bad habits."

If you really want a spot-free, well proportioned body you have to make a firm commitment. Your whole life is tied to what you eat. If you follow the program, I guarantee you will discover a wonderful new sense of self!

Disc jockey Casey Kasem looks younger today at 50 than he did at 25. He knows all too well that you are what you eat. He says about the Spot Reducing Diet, "It's like walking into some kind of gold mine. I think that what people find hardest to believe is that you can stop all your bad habits and still enjoy food and even enjoy it more. People are always looking for the easy way out. They ask Jean [Casey's wife] and me what they can and cannot eat on the program. We start to tell them and they say, 'That's a great diet.' And we say, 'It's not a diet. It's just rearranging the things you're eating so they work for you and eliminating the things that are the killers.' It doesn't take long to look and feel better."

Something for Everyone

Dr. Steven Shapiro, a Los Angeles pediatrician, came to me to learn how to increase his energy level. In the process of changing his eating habits he realized that the Spot Reducing Diet could benefit anyone who was motivated to lose weight slowly and sensibly. "To be quite honest," Dr. Shapiro says, "if everyone in this country followed the Spot Reducing Diet, we would have no more obesity. The program doesn't require a great deal of expense on the part of the individual. You can buy the food in any supermarket. It's just a shame that more people aren't motivated along these lines. You see, weight loss is motivation. If you're goal-oriented or motivated you can lose weight and if you reeducate your eating habits, then you can keep it off. That's what's so nice about this program. I don't foresee myself changing back to my old style of eating."

2

HOW TO BE A SUCCESSFUL DIETER

Dr. Richard Mettel sums up my sentiments when he says, "When you talk about losing weight, there is no such thing as a *miracle*. I have often dieted but this is the first time I have kept the weight off. That's the best part!"

Nearly three years ago Dr. Mettel joined my program and lost 30 pounds in about three and a half months. He became a successful dieter because he knew that the only way effectively to lose weight and keep it off is to do it slowly. For him, losing weight *in the right spots* came as a revelation.

"You want to lose weight fast," he says, "but you shouldn't. When you do, you're not losing fat, you're losing protein and water. If you think you're losing too slowly, then you'll never be able to lose it and keep it off. The most important thing, what makes a dieter successful, is changing his eating habits."

When Suzanne Somers came to me nearly ten years ago, she was 20 pounds heavier than she is today. "I'm a small-boned person," she says, "so I came to accept myself as being a little chunky. My mother's a little overweight and I thought that I had inherited the tendency. Then I lost a part on 'Starsky and Hutch,' and that really affected me. It was at the beginning of my career when a guest starring role meant a lot! I couldn't have been more excited about it.

". . . I was home learning the part and the day before I was supposed to show up on the set the producer called me and said, 'Suzanne, I hate to be the one to do this but we've been sitting around talking about it and you're just a little too chunky for the part.' I heard the word 'chunky' in association with me and I was devastated. I knew right then that I had to do something about the way I looked."

Instead of feeling sorry for herself, Suzanne made a commitment to get herself in shape. She began an exercise program with Ron Fletcher, and after her husband, Alan Hamel, became one of my clients she decided that achieving her physical goal had to be a combination of both diet and exercise.

Suzanne wanted to slim down all over but specifically she wanted to eliminate her saddlebags and slim down in the hips. In order to get in touch with her whole body it was essential for her to know exactly where she was out of proportion. And, second, to visualize how she would look with a perfect figure.

Most of my clients say, "Hermien, I don't like the way I look. I feel ugly so when I pass a mirror I just don't look. To be honest, I really don't know what I look like." This applies to young people as well as middle-aged and older. They don't like the way they look so they separate their heads from their bodies. If they feel like eating a carton of ice cream, they do. Or if they feel like drinking a few beers, they do. They have long since blocked the reality of "you are what you eat."

Take your clothes off and stand naked in front of a full-length mirror. See yourself the way you really are. Identify the spot or spots that you want to change and make a definite commitment to change them.

As we all know, Suzanne made the commitment and along with her husband switched from gourmet French cooking to my low-calorie recipes. They learned new eating habits while they were both hitting their spots. Suzanne went on to become one of America's favorite comediennes in the hit TV series "Three's Company." "I've never looked back," she says now. "Both Alan and I have made Hermien's program a way of life. And with each year that passes I know that I'm in control of my body, so the thought of aging doesn't threaten me. Eating properly is the best form of preventive medicine. I think when I'm 80 or 90 I'll still have a good figure."

Be patient!

It usually takes about a month to see a change in your shape. People will say, "Hermien, I don't know what's happened to me, I've lost only three pounds but my whole body's changed." It may take two weeks or two months, depending on which spot you're trimming. Everybody is different. Give yourself realistic expectations. Don't put too much faith in the scale. If you reach a plateau, don't think you've reached the end of the road; you're only in a traffic jam. Sometimes you may stay at the same weight for one to two weeks. When you are not losing weight—if you're doing everything you should—that is when your body is changing shape, redistributing weight.

The trick to losing weight and keeping it off is making certain conscious choices like: "I like myself better this way." Give yourself real incentive. If a shirt is too tight or a pair of jeans won't zip, it's thrilling when you are able to put them on and they fit perfectly. Some of my clients prefer taking their measurements once a week with a tape measure, while others prefer to monitor their spots using articles of clothing. Find the method that works best for you and use it.

Social Eating and Drinking

Once you know which foods fall into the carbohydrate, protein, and fat categories, you will know exactly what to expect when a waiter approaches you with a tray of hors d'oeuvres or when you approach a buffet table. You will ask yourself which foods are good for you and which ones aren't. If there's a doubt about it—don't eat it. Be your own best friend. Before you reach out for the petite pastry shell filled with mushrooms in *pesto* sauce, think about how you're going to feel the next day. The next day the champagne's gone, the beers are gone, the magic's gone, the people are gone, the thrill is gone, but the food and drink are not gone. They're on you. *If you eat it, you wear it.* You will learn that too much carbohydrate and fat are for that person, not this person. When you have trimmed your spots you will be able to be less regimented and still maintain your svelte shape.

I've had clients who could have one drink a day and lose weight while I've had others who would gain two pounds if they had one drink a week. You have to find out how much you can have. If drinking is a problem, if it's a big part of your life, give it up altogether while you're on the base program. (To counteract withdrawal symptoms see Sugar Withdrawal, p.25.)

If you're a social drinker you have several choices. The most obvious is *be less social for a few days or weeks, if necessary*. Give yourself a head start. Don't throw yourself at temptation's door. Go camping, read a book, chew sugarless gum, watch TV, start a new hobby. Change your pattern, and in doing so help yourself change your behavior. Eat and drink what *you* want, not what your friends and business associates want you to.

If lunch and dinner mean eating at a restaurant with people who will be drinking and will expect you to drink with them, order a nonalcoholic drink—a Virgin Mary instead of a Bloody Mary, Perrier instead of wine, or coffee instead of beer. Be proud of yourself for looking out for number one. Don't be embarrassed and don't feel sorry for yourself. The same goes for food. Actress Julie Carmen was feeling blue so she decided to console herself with a sweet treat. "I went to Famous Amos and said I'd like two cookies and a cup of coffee. They said they sold them only by the half pound, so I took a half pound. I ate the whole thing (when I used to go overboard, I *really* went overboard). I'm too much of a sugar addict to have a *little* sugar or a *little* cake or a *few* cookies. So I don't go near it. Now, however, I can go into a bakery and buy things I used to crave, for my guests, without feeling the slightest bit deprived. Having a perfect figure is my best reward."

If you make up your mind to give up a food that you love, the longer you are away from it the less you will crave it. Eventually you'll not even want it. And if you do want it, and if you can control it, you can have it!

My Maintenance Program will teach you how to eat and drink without getting your spots back or developing new ones. You can't go back to your old eating habits or you'll look the way you do now. You'll have to use the knowledge you've learned to keep yourself in shape.

The Baby-Food Taster

You have a new baby and you want to make sure that the food is tasty and just the right temperature. Smell and touch will have to tell you all you need to know—otherwise, you're going to keep gaining weight along with the baby.

The Gourmet-Cook Taster

Did you know that you can gain ten pounds in one week from *tasting*? That's right. If you can't control yourself when you're around food, when you're in the kitchen, or when you're in a friend's kitchen; if you suffer from hand-to-mouth disease, you will have to use ingenuity to lick the problem. Put surgical tape over your mouth while you're cooking. It won't hurt and it will hurt even less when you realize how it's saving you from eating hundreds of calories.

Hand-to-mouth disease is a very common problem. It's a habit that must be broken if you're going to be a successful dieter. And once you've lost weight you don't want to keep shoveling food into your mouth to see if it tastes right. *Use your nose.* If the cake batter smells good it will probably taste good too. Just because you're on a diet, that doesn't mean everyone else in the family has to be. They may not need to or want to lose weight. You're going to have to be your own best friend. Breaking the fattening habit of tasting as you cook is going to make a big difference to the size and shape of your spots.

The Midnight Eater and the TV Snacker

Both of you know who you are and which foods contributed to your midriff bulge or your saddlebags or your puffy face.

If you are a midnight eater, if you can't go to sleep on an empty stomach, *save one piece of fruit for bedtime.* When you eat a carbohydrate by itself you will experience a surge of energy followed by a rapid fall to exhaustion. Eating a piece of fruit before bedtime can become a permanent good habit.

If you like to snack in front of the TV, make sure you're snacking on something that's not going to compound your problem. If you're used to drinking wine, lots of fruit juice (one glass of orange juice is equal to eating three oranges), or soft drinks, make a trade. Drink mineral water, bouillon, herb tea, coffee, or ice water with lemon or lime. If you have to put something in your mouth while watching TV, make sure it's something that carries vitamins and minerals.

Eat raw vegetables instead of cake. See the recipe chapter for snack suggestions.

"Oh, I Never Eat a Meal, I Just Eat All Day"

If you can't stop eating but at the same time want to lose weight you will have a more difficult time, because you don't want to face a table with a place setting and a plate of food. You want food within reach at all times. If you're at your desk you eat cookies, pretzels, candies, and chips, or you drink soft drinks all day. You're never hungry at mealtime because you've been eating all day.

Whatever the reason, whatever your environment and lifestyle, if you recognize yourself, know that you can change your behavioral patterns and in doing so reshape your body. Plan to begin by eating six small meals a day. You won't feel deprived. Plan your meals. Make sure you are eating a balanced diet. I've designed the Spot Reducing Diet so that you can follow a daily regimen or create your own menus.

If you need to touch something, use worry beads. Use anything, but keep your hands away from food. And keep food out of sight until mealtimes.

The Closet Eater

You don't appear to overeat and yet you have lumps and bumps. Well, like a good little squirrel, you've developed the habit of hiding your cookies, candy, chips, nuts, and maybe even your wine and alcohol. You know that you shouldn't really be eating or drinking these things, so you do it secretly. You do it in private but you wear it in public. The answer for you is to empty those closets and drawers. Get rid of the hidden treats forever. Don't tempt yourself. Be your own best friend. You can't hide spots.

The Fat-Cell Count

Once you've been overweight you will always have the potential for being overweight again. It is as if your brain has a very fine computer chip that records how many fat cells you have had at any one time. If you had a paunchy stomach you will have to be aware of how easy it is to refill those "empty" fat cells. When you lose weight you empty them. But they're waiting . . . just like hungry, dry sponges they are always ready to fill up at a few days' notice. You will always be *reformed*, never cured. A *fat addict* will always be a fat addict and a *sugar addict* will always be a sugar addict. If you understand your problem and know how to control it, you will be able to save yourself from the repeated trials and nightmares of sugar and fat withdrawal.

Playing Chess with Food

You can have apple pie and cheese and remain within a certain caloric limit—you can be well fed but not well nourished. My objective is to give you the foundation upon which to build good, balanced eating habits. Just as the expert chess player plans his winning strategy, you will learn how to plan your diet strategically. Know which foods fall into the three basic categories and you'll find yourself making selections based on how your whole body will be affected.

In chess each piece has a certain value and a special way of moving. A bishop, for example, can move only along the diagonals of the chessboard, keeping only to the color from which it started—black or white. A knight can move two squares up and one to one side, jumping over other pieces if necessary. Think of each chess piece and its pattern of movement as you would think of foods and the spots on your body. If you are trying to lose your midriff bulge, are you willing to limit your wine intake to one four-ounce glass and omit your bread for that day? If saddlebags are your nemesis, will you select a bowl of strawberries—no cream—over chocolate mousse? If you know which spots specific foods and beverages affect, you will develop good food strategy.

In chess each move, each loss, each gain is clear. Not so with food. You are playing with, as well as against, yourself. The more you play the game, the more in control you become with each component piece—singly and in coordination with each other. Therefore you must learn the value or spot-producing potential of foods and likewise manipulate them within the strategy of your own diet plan. These values—read about what causes your spots—must

The Basics

be kept constantly in mind or the body will become out of proportion and, therefore, checkmated.

I don't want you counting calories. I want you to familiarize yourself with which foods fall into the carbohydrate, protein, and fat categories. Which ones *you* eat more than others—which ones caused your imbalances and which ones you have to learn to control. Once you learn to play chess with food you will be in control of not only your weight but your shape as well. If you eat or drink too much you'll know how to undo the damage before it's too late. Good food choices will become automatic. In my own case, if I eat half a can of unsalted peanuts I gain two pounds and half an inch in each of my thighs. If I eat an eighth of a can, nothing happens to me. Remember that you can have two different shapes at the same weight. If you want a well-balanced shape you must become adept at playing chess with food.

Ed McMahon tells a wonderful story about how playing chess with food saved his wife, Victoria, from being terribly disappointed on her birthday.

"Every year on Victoria's birthday at exactly 10:23 in the morning, the time she was born, I come in with Cristal champagne, caviar, sliced cucumbers, chopped egg yolk, the onions, and so forth. We were down at our place in Florida; it's very rural. We don't even have a mailbox, we have to go to the post office. But somehow on a Thursday—Victoria's birthday was on Saturday—I got seven ounces of the best Russian caviar sent to me from Ma Maison. How the UPS man found me I'll never know, but he did. I took the caviar out of the dry ice and I hid it behind the chicken and milk and Coca-Cola bottles in the refrigerator. I was secretly thrilled because I was all ready for Saturday.

"That night Victoria said, 'Oh, I'm so sick.' And I said, 'What's the matter?' And she said, 'My birthday's coming up and I can't have my caviar—it's not allowed and it's just going to wreck my day.' 'Oh, come on,' I said, 'it's your birthday!' 'Oh, no,' she said, 'I won't break for one day.' I have to admit she did look fantastic, but even so . . . The next morning I called Hermien in Los Angeles and told her the problem. She said, 'All right, just tell her to give up her bread and butter for today and tomorrow. She can have two ounces of caviar and one four-ounce glass of champagne.' So when I came in, Victoria started protesting, saying, 'No, I can't! I told you I can't.' But I said, 'I cleared it with Hermien Lee. She said it's fine as long as you give up your bread and butter today and tomorrow.' "

Victoria had mentioned caviar and champagne before she and Ed left for Florida and I told her to eat shrimp or crab and to drink only one four-ounce glass of dry white wine. Fortunately, Ed was clever enough to remember my theory of playing chess. When he called I knew that it meant so much to both of them to celebrate the way they had been celebrating for years. Everybody was happy. Victoria had her caviar and champagne and still hit her spots. The better your food sense, the easier and more fun playing chess will become.

Negative Energy

I've decided that the main reason people get fat is something I call *negative energy*. In the course of a day's work and emotions, people start to produce an emotional energy that continues to build—and they don't know where to put it. Because we're taught not to scream and not to carry on, we don't have an outlet for it. Often we can't get rid of this negative energy, so we eat. We stuff our faces until we're ready for bed and yet another day in which to continue the cycle.

There are two effective ways to handle negative energy: *activity* and *creativity*. By activity, I mean physical activity, exercise. Consider the full range, from walking at a fast pace to tap dancing. The important thing is to move your parts vigorously. I prefer exercising in the evening because it helps me to get rid of the day's frustrations, but I understand everyone has different rhythms. Exercise alone or with others. If you find yourself confined to your house or apartment at the end of the day, there are many good records, tapes, and cassettes to guide you through a routine.

Creativity isn't a substitute for activity, but it also works wonders. Getting lost in something you enjoy, something that makes your heart happy, provides a special sense of nourishment that food can't fulfill. That's why I encourage my clients to do something creative; for example, painting, woodworking, writing, sculpting, just about anything except gourmet cooking.

Once you are able to get rid of negative energy, you experience a lovely, quiet peace. You should have something around to eat, but make sure it's something you *may* eat, like a piece of fruit and partial skim milk cheese and a diet drink; your blood sugar may get too low otherwise.

Avoid Hidden Hunger

Over the years I have watched a pattern emerge that I call *hidden hunger*. This results when people make a habit of going from deprivation to reward: depriving themselves of nutritious food so that they can rationalize eating foods that contain mostly empty calories. They are bad chess players; believing that they must leave something off for fear of gaining weight, they choose to eat foods lacking in vitamins and minerals. Most of my clients don't even know that they're doing it.

Once their bad food choices are brought to light they see how to control their cravings. Usually what they've left out is some of their fruit or vegetable allotment. In one day, by going back on the program, they become able to overcome their seemingly irrational cravings.

This is one reason I stress meeting your daily spot-reducing requirements as well as taking a daily multivitamin with a mineral supplement. Occasionally, hidden hunger can be emotional. When things happen that affect you emotionally, it's even more important to eat properly; otherwise you will miss some necessary nutrients. You're depriving your body of something; but unfortunately, your conscious mind can't tell what it is. You develop cravings—which typically leads to reaching for those foods that exacerbate rather than solve the problem.

If you're under a lot of pressure or feeling particularly emotional, make sure that you have a good supply of nutritious food on hand. Balance your nutrients—don't undereat or overeat—and you'll help balance your emotions.

THE MASTER PLAN

3

THE SPOT REDUCING MASTER PLAN PROGRAM

Daily Requirements for Men and Women

PROTEIN

5'8" and taller	10 oz.
5'4½" to 5'8"	9 oz.
5'4" and shorter	8 oz.

3 cups of vegetables (refer to Vegetable Exchange List, p. 52)
3 servings of fruit (refer to Fruit Exchange List, p. 53)
2 slices of regular or 4 slices of very thin sliced whole wheat or rye bread
2 teaspoons of regular fat (for example, butter, oil, regular margarine, or mayonnaise) or 3 teaspoons of diet margarine
People who are 5'10" and taller may have an additional teaspoon of fat or margarine.

NOTE: If you lose more than 1½ pounds a week after the first week and you are under 5'4" you may have 9 oz. of protein instead of 8.

YOU WILL NEED:

bathroom scale
tape measure

food scale
measuring cup
measuring spoons
(If you don't have them, buy them!)

1. The bathroom scale is going to put you in touch with yourself. Weighing yourself should become as automatic as brushing your teeth. Don't be afraid of it. Use it as a tool. It will help you achieve your goal and maintain it.
2. The tape measure will help you monitor how your spots are disappearing or, heaven forbid!, reappearing. See Chapter 21 for measuring instructions.
3. The food scale is essential. It will teach you to judge the weight of fish, meat, poultry, and other food. Once you've become adept at guessing how much something weighs you'll be able to weigh your food visually.
4. Measuring cups will make you aware of exactly how much a half cup is in relation to a cup. What do three cups of vegetables really look like? Again, once you've been measuring things for a few weeks you'll be able to *eyeball* what you're served and know how much you're getting. This helps you develop good food sense.
5. Measuring spoons are important for the same reason as measuring cups. They are also essential tools for cooking. See the recipes in Chapter 14.

Food Chart

All my clients begin the program by filling in the answers to each column of the food chart on a daily basis. This enables them to get in touch with the way they eat. You may be amazed at what, when, and why you eat the way you do. There is a reason for your spots—it won't take you very long to find out what it is.

DATE AND DAY OF THE WEEK

Begin by writing down the date and the day of the week. That will make it easy to analyze your daily patterns.

TIME OF DAY

It is important to note what time you eat because most people don't know *when* they consume the most food. Some people never sit

DATE DAY OF WEEK	TIME OF DAY	AMOUNT & NAME OF FOOD	PLACE	WITH WHOM	WHAT'S HAPPENING	FEELINGS

down to a meal, they just eat all day. Some are unconscious eaters whose mouths chew right along with the television.

Many people believe that eating at night will make them gain weight or prevent them from losing it. I don't agree. In fact, I have my breakfast at midnight because if I eat breakfast in the morning I'm hungry all day.

Your body works all the time, even when you're asleep. If you eat less than the calories you burn, you're going to lose weight, and if you eat more, you're going to gain weight. It's as simple as that. It's what you consume in a 24-hour period that counts. What's most important is getting in touch with your body, listening to it, knowing when you need food the most and planning for those occasions. If you need breakfast, great! Eat it. If you like to eat before going to bed, that's okay, too, as long as you stay within your daily allotment.

AMOUNT AND NAME OF FOOD

The reason you must write down the amount and the kind of food and drink you consume is so that you will:

a. See what you consume, and the exact amounts.
b. Begin to develop good food sense. In a very few weeks you will be able to taste food and know whether or not it is loaded with hidden ingredients such as salt, butter, oil, or flour.

PLACE

Where you eat—at home, in a restaurant, at a friend's house—can make a difference in the amount of food you eat and how much you drink.

WITH WHOM

Do you eat more when you're alone or when you're with others?

WHAT'S HAPPENING?

Are you concentrating on eating or are you eating while concentrating on something else? Are you watching television? Are you at work? At a party? At the table? Learn to identify your habits.

FEELINGS AND FOOD DESIRES

Are you hungry? Are you angry? Frustrated? Learn the emotional cues that trigger your food habits. Because you are writing everything down you will undoubtedly stop yourself before consuming something you know you shouldn't. Write it down. Suppose you are tempted by a bowl of peanuts and you have to count them. You count out your six peanuts and because you have to stop, it makes you angry. Take the anger out by writing down what you really wanted. If you wanted 300 write it down in this column.

Master Plan Advice

You must eat *everything* on the daily Master Plan *every day*. Never cut down on anything, because you will upset the balance of the program. You may lose weight but unless you follow the

Master Plan *exactly* you won't lose it where you want it.

If you find that you aren't losing weight you may leave your bread off for a few days.

If you plan your own menus, always have at least two ounces of protein at lunch. I don't care how you meet your daily Master Plan requirements as long as you always have lunch.

If you wish to make your own menus, try using the Master Plan Guide.

For your convenience I have planned a month of deliciously balanced menus. Please use the exchange lists freely to insure variety. There is nothing boring about the Spot Reducing Diet. Especially if you use your imagination along with the menus!

Ground Rules

GENERAL

1. Take a good look at yourself in the nude. Know which spots you want to hit. Visualize how you want to look when you are finished with the program and are ready for the Maintenance Program.
2. Plan ahead—begin the program with a well stocked refrigerator and all the right tools.
3. Weigh yourself every morning but don't panic if you gain a pound or two or if you reach a plateau for a week or two.
4. Write down everything you eat and drink while you are on the base program.
5. Be sure you eat *all* your daily requirements—every day. If you go off the program, don't punish yourself by bingeing or starving. Simply continue the program.
6. Don't allow yourself to become bored. Play chess with food. Use the food-substitution lists.
7. Be sure to weigh and measure everything you eat until you are able to judge amounts just by looking.
8. *Exercise.* Even five minutes a day is better than nothing. Exercise is an appetite deterrent, and it will make you lose your spots faster.
9. Snack at the same time every day. By doing so you will help reset your appestat.
10. Develop good food sense.

11. Find ways to reward or console yourself other than by eating or drinking.
12. Be patient! Think of two months in relation to the rest of your life. If you want to have a sensational body, you have to allot two short months to purist activity—and while you're hitting your spots you are also learning new eating habits and a whole new nutritional vocabulary. Following this diet is the same as taking a short course in nutrition. You will be able to make better decisions based on your new knowledge.

Remember: when you are ready for the Maintenance Program you can eat anything you can control.

FOR THE SINGLE DIETER

1. Keep a pot of Hit the Spot vegetable soup or ratatouille on hand. You can always make a large amount and freeze some. I have eleven-year-old clients who do it.
2. Make two or three dinner dishes at a time, such as chicken breasts or Beverly Hills goulash, so that you will always have a good Hit the Spot meal waiting for you.
3. Make sure you always have foods you are allowed in the house. It's both easy and sensible to keep a few cans of tuna packed in water, partial skim milk cheese, frozen or canned vegetables in reserve.
4. Never forego a meal because you're too tired. You might begin to experience hidden hunger, and become caught in its trap.

FOR THE FAMILY

1. Ask your spouse to go on the program with you. Couples have a great advantage when they help each other.
2. If you know your family will balk at a low-calorie diet dish, no matter how delicious it tastes, don't tell them. The chances are they will never guess.
3. If your family makes you feel like the Lone Ranger, make up your own Hit the Spot dishes, divide them into single portions and freeze.

BEHAVIOR MODIFICATION

1. Never eat standing up.
2. Never eat in front of the refrigerator.

3. Never lick cooking spoons or taste food when cooking. Learn to rely on your sense of smell.
4. Never eat when you're reading or watching television. (This may be difficult, but you must do it.)
5. Put a place mat and utensils down, eat your meal, then put them away again.
6. When you take a bite of food, put your fork on your plate, your hands in your lap, taste and swallow the bite, then start over.
7. Never eat or drink when you're on the telephone.
8. Never taste anything from someone else's plate.
9. Never go to the market when you're hungry.
10. When having a salad in a restaurant, order Italian, French, or herb dressing on the side. Never order a dressing made with mayonnaise or blue cheese.

Hit the Spot Master Plan Guide

For breakfast make one selection from A, B, and C.
For lunch make one selection from D and E.
For the afternoon snack select one serving of fruit (see Fruit Exchange List, p. 53) and make one selection from group F.
For dinner make one selection from G and H. Include a hot vegetable (I) and a mixed vegetable salad (J).
See the recipe chapter for preparation directions.

BREAKFAST: A—1 orange
½ grapefruit
B—1 egg
1 oz. partial skim milk cheese
⅓ cup plain lowfat yogurt
1 T. specially prepared peanut butter
½ cup nonfat milk
C—1 scooped-out bagel (see p. 78)
1 slice regular whole wheat or rye bread
2 slices very thin sliced bread
½ cup cereal
coffee or tea

LUNCH: D—2 or 3 oz. tuna, chicken, turkey, crab, shrimp, chef salad without ham, egg salad, or lowfat cottage cheese
E—1 cup vegetables
coffee, tea, or diet soft drink

AFTERNOON SNACK: F—1 oz. protein, such as 1 T. specially prepared peanut butter
1 oz. partial skim milk cheese
⅓ cup lowfat cottage cheese
⅓ cup plain lowfat yogurt
1 oz. of any allowed protein

DINNER: G—4 or 5 oz. meat, fish, or poultry (red meat should be eaten only twice a week)
H—1 small baked or boiled potato
2 slices very thin sliced bread (if you don't have it now, you can have it before going to bed or at afternoon snack)
I—Hot vegetable or Hit the Spot vegetable soup (recipe on p. 141)
J—mixed vegetable salad

BEDTIME SNACK: K—1 serving of fresh fruit

NOTE: You may have 3 teaspoons of diet margarine or 2 teaspoons of regular fat a day (i.e., mayonnaise, butter, or regular margarine or oil). See the Exchange Lists. I also recommend drinking 8 8-oz. glasses of water each day.

Exchange Lists

VEGETABLES

(Vegetables marked with an asterisk have high vitamin A value. At least one serving of a high-A vegetable should be included in the diet each day.)

artichokes	brussel sprouts	chicory*
asparagus	cabbage	collards
beans, string, young	cauliflower	cucumbers
beet greens	celery	dandelion
broccoli	chard Swiss*	eggplant

escarole	mustard	spinach
greens	okra	summer squash
kale	pepper*	tomatoes*
lettuce	radishes	turnip greens
mushrooms	sauerkraut	watercress*

The following are higher in carbohydrate, so do not include more than ½ cup per day.

beets	onions	snow peas
carrots	peas, green	turnip
jicama	pumpkin*	winter squash*
	rutabaga	

The following are starchy vegetables and have more sugar value than the above. Eat them as you would bread.

corn	parsnips
corn on the cob	yam or sweet
lima beans	potato

FRUIT

(Fruits marked with an asterisk are rich sources of vitamin C (ascorbic acid). At least one serving should be included in the diet each day.)

Carbohydrate—10 grams per serving.

apple (2″)	1
applesauce (unsweetened)	½ cup
apricots—fresh	medium
dried	4 halves
banana	½ small
blackberries	1 cup
blueberries	½ cup
cantaloupe (6″)*	¼ slice
cherries	10 large
dates	2
figs	2
figs—fresh	2 large
dried	1 small
grapefruit*	½ small

grapes	12
honeydew melon (7")	1/8 slice
mango	1/2 small
orange*	1 small
papaya	1/3 cup
peach	1 medium
pear	1 small
pineapple	1/2 cup or 2 slices
plums	2 medium
prunes—dried	2 medium
raisins	2 teaspoons
raspberries	1 cup
strawberries*	1 cup
tangerine*	1 large
watermelon	1 cup

Unsweetened canned fruits may be used in the same amounts as listed for the fresh fruits. Make sure the label says "in water" or "in its own juice."

BREAD AND STARCH

bread

scooped bagel	equals	1 slice bread
biscuit, roll (2")		1 " "
muffin (2")		1 " "
corn bread (1/2" cube)		1 " "
flour		2½T.

cereal

cooked	1/2 cup
dry	1/2 cup
rice and grits, cooked	1/2 cup
spaghetti and noodles, cooked	1/2 cup

crackers

graham (2½" sq.)	2
Oysterettes	20
soda (2½" sq.)	2
saltines (2" sq.)	5
round thin (1½")	6-8

vegetables
 beans and peas, dried cooked
  (lima, navy, split peas &
  cowpeas) — ½ cup
  lima beans, fresh — ½ cup
  baked beans, no pork — ¼ cup
corn
 sweet, fresh — 1 small or ½ large
 popped — ⅓ cup
parsnips — 1 cup
potatoes, white
 baked — 1
 boiled, 2" — 1
 mashed — ½ cup
sweet potatoes or yams — ¼ cup

One regular slice of bread is equal to 2 slices of very thin sliced bread.

PROTEIN

Remove the fat, skin and bones before weighing meat, fish, or poultry.

1 oz. of meat = 1 protein substitute.

chicken, white meat only	1 oz.
meat, medium fat (beef, lamb, liver)	1 oz.
fish	
cod	1 oz.
tuna packed in water	1 oz.
crab	1 oz.
oysters, shrimp, clams	
(NOTE: See Fat and Lean Fish list for other choices.)	
frankfurters (8 or 9 per pound)*	1
cheese (see Cheese Exchange List, p. 56)	
American	¾ oz.

*Frankfurters are high in fat and should not be eaten more than once a month during the *base* diet.

cottage	⅓ cup lowfat
egg	1
peanut butter*	1 T.
yogurt	⅓ cup plain lowfat

NOTE: To substitute milk for protein:
1 cup of nonfat milk equals 1 ounce of meat. A *maximum* of 1 cup a day is allowed.

FAT

butter or diet margarine	1 t.
cream, light 20%	2 T.
heavy 40%	1 T.
cream cheese	1 T.
French dressing	1 T.
mayonnaise	1 t.
oil or cooking fat	1 t.
nuts	6 small
olives	5 small
avocado (4″)	⅛ inch slice
peanut butter	1 t.

CHEESE

¾ oz. of hard cheese = 1 oz. of partial skim milk cheese

HARD	PARTIAL SKIM MILK
jack	mozzarella or string
Muenster	Lite Line: American, Swiss, cheddar, or jack
Swiss	Weight Watchers
American	Laughing Cow Green Label:

*Peanut butter must be old-fashioned or natural style (oil floating on top) and the oil must be removed continuously throughout the duration of the jar. Instead of appearing oily, it should look flat (matte). When the oil is removed, the peanut butter will become dry and crunchy. You will enjoy a very satisfying texture and taste. One tablespoon a day will provide a treat as well as a burst of energy when coupled with a carbohydrate such as an apple.

Jarlsberg (1¼ wedge for 1 oz. protein or
Parmesan 1 wedge + 1 cube.
6 small cubes = 1 oz. protein)

Only 1 ounce of partial skim milk cheese or ¾ oz. hard cheese per day.

Do not eat cheddar cheese until you've finished the program.

NOTE: For cottage cheese, see Protein Exchange List, p. 55.

Following are examples of cheeses which you may not eat until you are on Maintenance:
 Brie, Camembert, triple creme, Gorgonzola, blue, or Roquefort.

4

A SPOT REDUCING MONTH OF MENUS

The month of menus has been prepared to show you that losing weight and learning good nutrition can be a delicious experience. The daily menus have been planned to add spice and variety to your life. There is nothing boring about the Spot Reducing Diet.

Use the Exchange Lists in conjunction with the daily menus or, if you want to, plan your own menus using the tools and recipes I've given you (see Chapter 14) and make sure you meet your daily requirements.

Bon appétit!

Monday

BREAKFAST: 1 orange or ½ grapefruit
1 egg, any style (be sure the white is well done)
1 slice whole wheat toast or 2 slices very thin sliced whole wheat toast
coffee or tea

LUNCH: 1 scoop tuna salad (see p. 148)
lettuce, tomato, green pepper, and mushrooms
diet dressing
coffee, tea, or diet soft drink

LATE AFTERNOON SNACK:	1 apple 1 T. specially prepared peanut butter
DINNER:	4 or 5 oz. roast chicken breast or turkey breast (never eat dark meat; see p. 154 for turkey breast in a bag) small baked potato steamed broccoli (see Vegetable Exchange List for substitution, p. 52) mixed green salad with diet dressing ("fork-prong" dressing; see p. 80)
BEDTIME SNACK:	⅓ medium cantaloupe or comparable fruit on the exchange list

Tuesday

BREAKFAST:	1 orange or ½ grapefruit 1 oz. partial skim milk string cheese (melted or hard) 1 slice whole wheat toast or 2 slices very thin sliced whole wheat toast or a scooped-out whole wheat bagel (see p. 78, for scooped-out bagels. Remember: Rye bread can be substituted for whole wheat bread.) coffee or tea Melting your string cheese on toast or inside a toasted, scooped whole wheat bagel is delicious.
LUNCH:	tomato stuffed with bay shrimp, or tuna or crab salad lettuce, cucumbers, and mushrooms with diet dressing coffee, tea, or diet soft drink

LATE AFTERNOON SNACK:	⅓ cup lowfat plain yogurt or lowfat cottage cheese 1 cup fresh strawberries (or use frozen, unsweetened)
DINNER:	baked halibut ⅓ cup cooked brown or wild rice 1 t. butter or diet margarine zucchini or summer squash
BEDTIME SNACK:	1 peach or comparable fruit—see Fruit Exchange List, p. 53

Wednesday

BREAKFAST:	½ cup shredded wheat ½ cup nonfat milk ½ banana coffee or tea
LUNCH:	2-egg spinach and cheese omelet (see Cheese Exchange List p. 56) sliced tomatoes 1 slice whole wheat toast or scooped whole wheat bagel coffee, tea, or diet soft drink Remember: when ordering an omelet in a restaurant, be sure to specify a *two-egg omelet* because most omelets are made with three eggs. If you have a cheese omelet, always have it made with a vegetable filler, because cheese has a lot of fat in it. A vegetable filler means that they won't overload you with cheese. Try spinach, zucchini, or broccoli.

LATE AFTERNOON SNACK:	⅓ cup lowfat cottage cheese or plain lowfat yogurt 1 orange
DINNER:	curried chicken (see p. 152) large vegetable salad with diet dressing green beans or broccoli potato skin (optional)
BEDTIME SNACK:	⅓ cantaloupe or comparable fruit

Thursday

BREAKFAST:	1 orange or ½ grapefruit 1 egg, any style (if it is fried or scrambled, use Pam) 1 slice whole wheat toast or 2 slices very thin sliced whole wheat toast or 1 scooped bagel—preferably whole wheat or rye 1 t. butter or diet margarine coffee or tea NOTE: If you're having a scrambled egg you may add one extra white.
LUNCH:	1 scoop tuna, turkey, or chicken salad sliced tomatoes, green pepper, red pepper Boston or romaine lettuce, green onions (optional) diet salad dressing coffee, tea, or diet soft drink
LATE AFTERNOON SNACK:	½ banana (great frozen) with 1 T. specially prepared peanut butter (see p. 79)

DINNER:	Beverly Hills goulash (see p. 158) mixed green salad with diet dressing steamed carrots
BEDTIME SNACK:	1 peach or comparable fruit

Friday

BREAKFAST:	1 orange or ½ grapefruit 1 oz. string cheese 1 slice whole wheat toast or 2 slices very thin sliced whole wheat toast or 1 scooped whole wheat bagel 1 t. butter or diet margarine coffee or tea NOTE: if you melt the cheese, save your fat allotment for lunch or dinner.
LUNCH:	breast of turkey 1 cup Hit the Spot cole slaw (see p. 148) In a restaurant you may have ½ cup cole slaw. sliced tomatoes and cucumbers coffee, tea, or diet soft drink
LATE AFTERNOON SNACK:	1 wedge plus 1 cube Laughing Cow Green Label cheese or slice of Lite Line cheese 1 apple
DINNER:	spicy fish fillets (see p. 150) ½ cup cooked brown or wild rice mixed vegetable salad broccoli, green beans, or zucchini
BEDTIME SNACK:	½ cup blueberries or comparable fruit

The Master Plan

Saturday

BREAKFAST: ⅓ cup plain lowfat yogurt or lowfat cottage cheese
1 cup fresh or frozen unsweetened strawberries
coffee or tea

LUNCH: 2 slices very thin sliced whole wheat bread
tuna salad, egg salad, shrimp salad or chicken salad (Make a sandwich, or if you're in a restaurant and you order a sandwich, either remove one slice of bread or eat the whole sandwich and count it as your starch for the day. You may have a potato *skin* with dinner if you want.)
sliced cucumbers
coffee, tea, or diet soft drink

LATE AFTERNOON SNACK: ½ banana with 1 T. specially prepared peanut butter

DINNER: lean leg of lamb or a lamb shoulder chop
large vegetable salad with diet dressing
steamed cauliflower or spinach or broccoli

BEDTIME SNACK: 1 orange

Sunday

BREAKFAST: Hit the Spot French toast (see p. 145)
coffee or tea

THE SPOT REDUCING DIET

LUNCH: chef salad (see p. 147) with diet dressing or regular dressing on the side (If you're in a restaurant remember: no ham, no cheese and three times as much turkey.)
⅓ of a cantaloupe or a comparable fruit
coffee, tea, or diet soft drink

LATE AFTERNOON SNACK: 1 apple and 1 wedge plus 1 cube of Laughing Cow Green Label cheese or 1 slice of Lite Line or 1 slice of Weight Watchers cheese

DINNER: veal loaf (see p. 157)
small baked potato
1 cup Hit the Spot ratatouille (see p. 159)
1 t. butter or diet margarine

BEDTIME SNACK: 1 pear or comparable fruit

Monday

BREAKFAST: 1 orange or ½ grapefruit
½ cup shredded wheat
½ cup nonfat milk
coffee or tea

LUNCH: 3 oz. cold veal loaf
sliced tomatoes and cucumbers with diet dressing
½ papaya
coffee, tea, or diet soft drink

LATE AFTERNOON SNACK: 1 T. specially prepared peanut butter
1 carrot and 1 stalk celery

The Master Plan

DINNER: Malibu tuna (see p. 149)
1 artichoke
1 t. diet margarine or butter
mixed vegetable salad with diet dressing

BEDTIME SNACK: strawberry cloud (see p. 144) or 1 cup strawberries

Tuesday

BREAKFAST: 1 small peach
½ cup puffed wheat or oatmeal
⅓ to ½ cup nonfat milk
coffee or tea

LUNCH: ½ small cantaloupe stuffed with crab salad on romaine or bibb lettuce
1 cup vegetable soup (if at home for lunch; if not, 1 cup other vegetables—see Vegetable Exchange List, p. 52)
coffee, tea, or diet soft drink

LATE AFTERNOON SNACK: 1 cup frozen unsweetened strawberries or 1 orange
⅓ cup plain lowfat yogurt

DINNER: marinated fish fillets—use bass, halibut, red snapper, or sole (see p. 150)
1 small baked potato
string beans and mushrooms
mixed vegetable salad

BEDTIME SNACK: 1 large scooped potato skin filled with chopped tomatoes, onions, and mustard, or see Vegetable Exchange List, p. 52
½ cup rhubarb dessert (see p. 162)

Wednesday

BREAKFAST: 1 orange or 1 tangelo
1 scrambled egg in Teflon pan with 1 extra egg white
1 slice whole wheat or rye toast or 2 slices very thin sliced whole wheat toast
1 t. butter or diet margarine
coffee or tea

LUNCH: tuna stuffed into a green pepper or tomato
cold asparagus or any vegetable
coffee, tea, or diet soft drink

LATE AFTERNOON SNACK: strawberry cloud
1 T. specially prepared peanut butter
If you are full, don't eat the peanut butter and add an extra ounce of protein at dinner

DINNER: soy chicken (see p. 154)
½ cup steamed brown rice
1 cut mixed cauliflower and broccoli
vegetable salad

BEDTIME SNACK: 1 oz. partial skim milk cheese
1 scooped potato skin

Thursday

BREAKFAST: ½ cup frozen or fresh blueberries without sugar or ½ banana
⅓ cup plain lowfat yogurt
coffee or tea

LUNCH:	2-egg spinach or zucchini cheese omelet; use mozzarella cheese if possible 1 scooped-out bagel 1 t. butter or diet margarine coffee, tea, or diet soft drink
LATE AFTERNOON SNACK:	1 small apple 1 T. specially prepared peanut butter
DINNER:	sliced turkey ½ cup cooked rice with a dash of milder soy (less salty) or Worcestershire sauce 1 cup steamed spinach, chopped with garlic and onions 1 cup ratatouille
BEDTIME SNACK:	strawberry cloud

Friday

BREAKFAST:	½ grapefruit ½ cup cooked oatmeal ½ cup nonfat milk coffee or tea
LUNCH:	bowl of vegetable soup ⅔ cup lowfat cottage cheese mixed with chopped onions, tomatoes, or green pepper; you can add mustard to cottage cheese if desired whole tomato coffee, tea, or diet soft drink
LATE AFTERNOON SNACK:	1 pear with 1 ounce of protein
DINNER:	hamburger (see p. 155) Hit the Spot potato chips (see p. 159) steamed broccoli sliced tomatoes and onions
BEDTIME SNACK:	1 serving fruit

Saturday

BREAKFAST:
1 orange
1 poached egg (make sure white is cooked hard, because soft egg white has a protein called avidin that makes biotin, part of the B complex, insoluble)
1 slice whole wheat toast or 2 slices very thin sliced whole wheat toast
1 t. butter or diet margarine
coffee or tea

LUNCH:
cold soy chicken breast or chicken salad
1 bowl vegetable soup—if at home; if not, see vegetable exchange list
sliced tomatoes, cucumbers, onions
coffee, tea, or diet soft drink

LATE AFTERNOON SNACK:
1 small apple
1 T. specially prepared peanut butter

DINNER:
4–5 oz. cooked shrimp in ratatouille over ½ cup steamed brown rice
mixed vegetable salad

BEDTIME SNACK:
1 serving fruit

Sunday

BRUNCH:
mixed melon cup: ¼ small cantaloupe with small slivers of honeydew
3 oz. chicken livers sauteed in dry vermouth
1 t. cream cheese (instead of fat)
1 scooped bagel
coffee or tea

The Master Plan

LATE AFTERNOON SNACK:	1 bowl of vegetable soup if desired ½ banana 1 T. specially prepared peanut butter
DINNER:	Chili con carne (see p. 155) with lean veal or leftover chicken or turkey 1 corn tortilla or ½ cup steamed brown rice raw celery, carrots, cauliflower, onions, green and red pepper, cut up and used as a salad or relish 1 serving fruit
BEDTIME SNACK:	1 potato skin with 1 t. butter or diet margarine

Monday

BREAKFAST:	⅓ medium cantaloupe ⅓ cup lowfat cottage cheese coffee or tea
LUNCH:	turkey sandwich made with 2 slices of very thin sliced whole wheat bread and sliced turkey tomato mustard lettuce dill pickle (wash and slice) 1 cup Hit the Spot cole slaw coffee, tea or diet soft drink
LATE AFTERNOON SNACK:	1 small apple 1 oz. partial skim milk cheese
DINNER:	veal stew (see p. 156) steamed broccoli red onion and sliced tomato salad ½ cup brown or wild rice

BEDTIME SNACK:	1 orange

Tuesday

BREAKFAST:	1 apple 1 T. specially prepared peanut butter coffee or tea
LUNCH:	tuna salad stuffed into a tomato 1 hard boiled egg *white* green pepper or any vegetable coffee, tea, or diet soft drink
LATE AFTERNOON SNACK:	½ small cantaloupe ⅓ cup lowfat cottage cheese
DINNER:	2 enchiladas (see p. 155) Hermien's hot tomato sauce (see p. 161) chopped vegetable salad
BEDTIME SNACK:	1 serving fruit

Wednesday

BREAKFAST:	1 orange egg in the nest coffee or tea 　Egg in the nest: Cut a hole in a piece of very thin sliced whole wheat bread with a biscuit cutter. Fry one side of bread in 1 teaspoon diet margarine, turn over, add egg to hole in bread, and fry that side.

LUNCH:	1 scooped bagel Add either 1 or 2 oz. of turkey plus 1 oz. partial skim milk cheese, chopped onions and chopped tomatoes, mustard; bake 10 minutes at 350°. 1 bowl vegetable soup coffee, tea, or diet soft drink
LATE AFTERNOON SNACK:	strawberry cloud or 1 apple and 1 oz. turkey breast (If you have the strawberry cloud, it counts as only 1 serving of fruit. If you have it you may add an extra ounce of protein at dinner or before bed.)
DINNER:	Marinated chicken breasts (see p. 139) ½ cup cooked brown rice chopped steamed spinach and mushrooms green salad
BEDTIME SNACK:	1 serving fruit

Thursday

BREAKFAST:	½ grapefruit ⅓ cup lowfat cottage cheese coffee or tea
LUNCH:	Spanish omelet (see p. 147) with or without 1 oz. cheese 1 bowl vegetable soup 1 slice whole wheat or rye toast or scooped bagel coffee, tea, or diet soft drink
LATE AFTERNOON SNACK:	½ banana 1 T. specially prepared peanut butter

DINNER:	Hit the Spot chicken Kiev (see p. 152) ½ cup cooked brown or wild rice steamed broccoli and cherry tomatoes vegetable salad
BEDTIME SNACK:	1 serving fruit

Friday

BREAKFAST:	1 cup frozen unsweetened strawberries ⅓ cup plain lowfat yogurt 1 slice regular whole wheat toast or 2 slices very thin sliced whole wheat toast or 1 scooped bagel coffee or tea
LUNCH:	cold leftover barbecued halibut raw vegetables salad with 1 t. mayonnaise; mayonnaise can be diluted with French's or Dijon mustard or water or vinegar or lemon juice (you may use one or all of these) coffee, tea, or diet soft drink
LATE AFTERNOON SNACK:	1 serving fruit and 1 oz. partial skim milk cheese
DINNER:	turkey breast in a bag 1 small baked potato ½ cup steamed carrots vegetable salad
BEDTIME SNACK:	1 serving fruit

The Master Plan

Saturday

BREAKFAST:	1 orange 2 slices Hit the Spot French toast (see p. 145) coffee or tea
LUNCH:	scoop of tuna, chicken, shrimp, or crab salad celery, carrots, radishes coffee, tea, or diet soft drink
LATE AFTERNOON SNACK:	1 pear and 1 T. specially prepared peanut butter
DINNER:	1 small fillet steak ½ cup cooked brown rice or 1 small baked potato hot vegetable mixed vegetable salad
BEDTIME SNACK:	1 serving fruit

Sunday

BRUNCH:	fresh fruit salad ⅔ cup lowfat cottage cheese 1 scooped bagel 1 t. butter or diet margarine coffee or tea
LATE AFTERNOON SNACK:	1 small apple 1 oz. partial skim milk cheese
DINNER:	chili con carne ½ cup cooked brown rice relishes
BEDTIME SNACK:	1 scooped potato skin chopped tomatoes, onions, and mustard

Monday

BREAKFAST:	1 orange or ½ grapefruit 1 poached egg on whole wheat toast or 1 soft-boiled egg (white well done) 1 t. butter or diet margarine coffee or tea
LUNCH:	⅔ cup lowfat cottage cheese mixed with green pepper, tomato, green onions, and a dash of Dijon or regular mustard coffee, tea, or diet soft drink
LATE AFTERNOON SNACK:	1 Laughing Cow Green Label cheese wedge plus 1 cube or 1 slice Lite Line or Weight Watchers cheese 1 serving fruit
DINNER:	spicy liver (see p. 156) ½ cup brown or wild rice vegetable soup or steamed mixed vegetables
BEDTIME SNACK:	1 cup strawberries

Tuesday

BREAKFAST:	½ cup shredded wheat ½ banana ½ cup nonfat milk coffee or tea
LUNCH:	salade Niçoise (see p. 148) coffee, tea, or diet soft drink
LATE AFTERNOON SNACK:	⅓ cup plain lowfat yogurt or lowfat cottage cheese 1 serving fruit
DINNER:	veal scallopini (see p. 157) ½ cup brown or wild rice steamed broccoli or zucchini

BEDTIME SNACK:
12 frozen grapes
NOTE: Grapes are high in sugar. Freezing them makes them go further and it allows you to savor their delicious flavor longer.

Wednesday

BREAKFAST:
½ cup cooked oatmeal
½ cup nonfat milk
1 orange
coffee or tea

LUNCH:
½ small papaya stuffed with bay shrimp salad
coffee, tea, or diet soft drink

LATE AFTERNOON SNACK:
1 hard-boiled egg
mixed vegetable salad

DINNER:
poached snapper (see p. 151)
Hit the Spot potato chips (see p. 159)
steamed broccoli, carrots, and cauliflower

BEDTIME SNACK:
1 serving fruit

Thursday

BREAKFAST:
Hit the Spot French toast
½ grapefruit
coffee or tea

LUNCH:
seafood or chicken salad
sliced tomatoes and cucumbers
coffee, tea, or diet soft drink

LATE AFTERNOON SNACK:
1 T. specially prepared peanut butter
½ banana

DINNER: 1 lamb chop (shoulder cut) or roast leg of lamb
small baked potato
spinach and onions (see p. 160)
1 t. butter or diet margarine

BEDTIME SNACK: ½ cup blueberries

Friday

BREAKFAST: 1 scooped bagel
1 oz. string cheese or 1 t. butter or diet margarine
coffee or tea

LUNCH: fresh fruit salad
⅔ cup lowfat cottage cheese
coffee, tea, or diet soft drink

LATE AFTERNOON SNACK: 1 oz. tuna
2 celery stalks
small mixed vegetable salad

DINNER: vegetable soup
soy chicken
steamed artichoke
1 t. butter or diet margarine

BEDTIME SNACK: 2 slices very thin sliced whole wheat bread
1 wedge Laughing Cow Green Label cheese or 1 slice partial skim milk cheese
sliced tomatoes and onions (optional)

Saturday

BREAKFAST: 1 T. specially prepared peanut butter
½ scooped bagel or 1 slice very thin sliced whole wheat or rye toast
½ grapefruit or 1 orange
coffee or tea

The Master Plan

LUNCH: chef salad (remember: three times the turkey and no ham or cheese)
½ scooped bagel
1 t. butter or diet margarine
coffee, tea, or diet soft drink

LATE AFTERNOON SNACK:
1 apple
1 wedge plus 1 cube Laughing Cow Green Label cheese

DINNER: bouillabaisse (see p. 140)
large mixed vegetable salad

BEDTIME SNACK: 1 serving fruit

Sunday

BRUNCH: tomato, mushroom, onion omelet (see p. 147)
2 slices very thin sliced whole wheat toast with ¾ oz. Parmesan cheese or comparable Hit the Spot cheese selection
fresh fruit compote
coffee or tea
NOTE: Fresh fruit compote: have one cup, as you are having fruit only twice today.

LATE AFTERNOON SNACK:
1 cup vegetable soup
1 oz. chicken breast or 1 oz. shrimp

DINNER: turkey breast in a bag (save 1 oz. protein for bedtime)
1 small baked potato
ratatouille
mixed vegetable salad

BEDTIME SNACK: ½ frozen banana with 1 T. specially prepared peanut butter

Hermien's Helpful Hints

1 scoop of tuna or chicken salad is equal to 3 oz. of protein in a restaurant. If it's loaded with mayonnaise, leave the 2 teaspoons of fat off your plan for that day. If the salad doesn't contain much mayonnaise, leave off 1 teaspoon of fat that day.

Eat everything on the Master Plan every day. You may leave the bread off if you want, but that is the only thing. If you leave your bread off and become constipated, take 3 tablespoons of Miller's bran a day.

Use only cereals that contain less than 5 percent sugar. For example: Shredded Wheat, Puffed Wheat or Puffed Rice, Oatmeal, Wheatena. Read labels.

Popcorn isn't such a bad food. It's the company it keeps that counts. Two cups of plain popped corn with no fat or salt is equal to one slice of bread. Get an air popper. Do not order popcorn at a movie because they pop it in oil.

If you want to use chewing gum, use Trident

Trident	4 calories per stick
Orbit	7 calories per stick
Carefree	8 calories per stick
Chewels	10 calories per stick

You may have one scooped-out bagel a day. It must be whole wheat or rye, never pumpernickel, which contains white flour and caramelized sugar. If you can't buy whole wheat or rye bagels, get egg or onion, though whole wheat and rye are more nutritious. Cut the bagel in two. Toast it. Take a knife and circle the rim by the hole and by the edge. Then take a spoon and remove the bread from the bagel. You're left with a deliciously crispy and highly satisfying crust.

The Master Plan

If you want additional fiber in your diet, have 3 heaping tablespoons of unprocessed bran a day. (Try Miller's bran.) Mix it with ½ cup applesauce (½ cup unsweetened is 1 fruit serving) or ⅓ cup of cottage cheese (that amount of cottage cheese equals 1 oz. of protein). Some people mix bran with water and a squeeze of lemon juice. Do not use regular processed bran; it contains too much sugar.

The following foods contain negligible amounts of carbohydrates, protein, and fat. Therefore they should be used as desired in the diet.

coffee	cranberries*	pickles, sour*†
tea	lemon	pickles, dill*†
clear broth	mustard	saccharin
bouillon	spices	pepper
potato skin (1 per day, skin only)	gelatin (unsweetened)	vinegar

Buy old-fashioned peanut butter or natural peanut butter. Be sure you can see oil resting on top of the peanut butter. Laura Scudder, Deaf Smith, or Skippy are examples of ones which are easy to prepare.

Remove the lid and pour the oil off the top of the jar. Wad up a paper towel, place on peanut butter inside the jar, replace the lid and turn upside down. If you can't close the lid, place the jar with paper towel inside upside down on a plate. *Do not put in the refrigerator.*

In 15 minutes that paper towel will be saturated with oil. Replace it with a clean towel. (Be sure to use a strong, absorbent paper towel.) Leave upside down another 15 minutes.

Remove towel, pierce peanut butter with a fork to get at the excess oil. Piercing it will also remove any air that might be in the peanut butter. Repeat the process: place a clean paper towel inside the jar, seal it and turn upside down. Always leave it out of the refrigerator.

Preparing your peanut butter usually takes one day. You must keep changing the paper towels—about five or six—until the peanut butter appears dull. If it's still shiny, but hard, pat with a paper

---

*You may include these as extras, but always in moderation.
†Pickles must be washed to remove salt.

towel and use. Repeat this process throughout the life of the jar. You will use approximately 25 paper towels.

If your peanut butter is dull, take a tablespoon and scoop out a level measurement. If the tablespoon of peanut butter is too hard or too dry for you to spread, place it in a bowl and add a small amount of water to it. Or heat it in a spoon. (Occasionally, when it's dry, you will have to use your fingers to get it out of the jar.)

Keep changing the paper towels for the duration of the jar. After removing a portion of peanut butter, stir the remainder and restuff the jar with clean paper towels. Always keep it upside down and out of the refrigerator.

Fork-prong it. Have you ever noticed how a salad arrives either glistening with oil or blanketed with a thick dressing? The thick, gloppy dressing doesn't generally sink to the bottom of the bowl—no, you eat it all. Very fattening! Oil and vinegar dressing glides over the vegetables and what you don't eat with your salad makes a nice little pool in the bottom of your bowl.

In either case, when you eat salad with dressing already on it, you're asking for far more calories than you need. You're eating fat, and fat is fattening. Even the so-called "light" dressings have far more oil than you need if you're going to spot reduce.

You must order your salad with dressing on the side and you must "fork-prong it." Dip your fork into Italian, French, or herb dressing (never a heavy creamy dressing), getting just enough to add a touch of flavor to your next bite of salad. What you will soon discover is that vegetables taste delicious without a thick, fattening disguise—you get a lot of taste and don't have to count it as anything.

When you do not fork-prong your dressing, don't have more than 16 calories a day of salad dressing. Read the label. Bernstein's low-calorie vinaigrette or low-calorie Italian with cheese has 2 calories per tablespoon, so you can have up to 8 tablespoons.

Here is a checklist to help you determine which varieties of beef you can safely enjoy—and which you must stay away from—while you are spot reducing:

The Master Plan

ALLOWED	NOT ALLOWED
steak: fillet top sirloin flank	steak: New York porterhouse T-bone
roasts: chateaubriand sirloin tip top of the round (lean)	roasts: prime rib tri tip
hamburger: round or top (not marbled)	hamburger in a package corned beef stew meat chuck brisket

REMEMBER: Only twice a week, if ever, of the "allowed" group. Do not eat pork except on Maintenance Program (see Chapter 21).

HIT THE SPOT!

5

THE FACE AND NECK

When a new client walks into my office, his or her eating habits are reflected by the tone and texture of the skin, the sheen and texture of the hair, and the brightness or dullness of the eyes. Your face is a mirror. It shows what's going on inside, and even with the aid of creams, lotions, hair conditioners, and makeup you can camouflage bad eating and drinking habits for only short periods of time. The only way to look beautiful or handsome naturally is to eat the correct balance of protein, fat, and carbohydrate. By rebalancing your nutrients you can make your skin reflect a healthy, radiant glow, your hair will look healthy and shiny, and your eyes will sparkle.

Losing Face—the Typical Dieter's Syndrome

On most diets, the first spot to lose weight is the face. You get that gaunt, puckered, drawn look. Dark circles may appear under your eyes, and your eyes may even look dull. There is a reason for it—and it's not simply because you're losing weight; it's because you're losing weight *too fast*.

One of the most important reasons to lose weight slowly is so you won't look emaciated and exhausted. When Casey Kasem came to me he was doing his weekly television show, "America's Top 10" and he wanted to avoid the typical dieter's syndrome. I told him he needed more protein in his diet. A vegetarian, he was getting too much carbohydrate for the protein and fat he was consuming. He wanted to lose ten pounds and increase his energy level without compromising his looks.

Casey told me, "Up until the time I went to you I had tried a variety of diets and I always had the same problem—either my cheeks would get thin or my neck or my chest, and I would just begin to look scrawny. People would say I wasn't looking good. But I've never had anybody tell me I wasn't looking good since I've been sticking by the Hermien method. At the same time that you're losing quickly, you don't lose it in your face, so you don't look as though you've been dieting or fasting for 12 straight days. That's probably the most exciting thing about the program. You look great after you start it and you just continue to look and feel better and better!"

Joy Philbin came to me to trim her saddlebags and was amazed when she was able to hit that specific spot without losing weight in her face. "My face didn't get thin," she says enthusiastically. "I didn't have that drawn, haggard look that you have when you diet. In fact, my eyes were much brighter. My skin tone was rosier. I didn't need as much makeup."

As you slowly lose weight your face will slowly change its shape. The roundness and puffiness will disappear. If you have a double chin, it will disappear. It's difficult to say how quickly this will happen but if you don't have much weight to lose you may be able to reshape your face in two weeks.

Your Complexion

If your face has a pasty, gray look, it's because you have what I call the *carbohydrate look*. Far too many carbohydrates, empty calories that don't carry vitamins and minerals—cookies, candy, soft drinks, even too much regular chewing gum—will give you this unhealthy look.

Balance your nutrients over a period of at least three weeks and the color will return to your face. There is something magic in vegetables. Like them or not, if you want to have beautiful skin you've got to eat them. Those garden-grown nutrients will help you lose weight without sagging, bagging, and wrinkling.

Too much fat over a long period of time can cause tiny white bumps that form beneath the eyes. They're fatty deposits that won't go away unless they're professionally removed.

Too much fat can also cause enlarged pores. This can be very unattractive, especially on a young person. Large pores can be made smaller if you rebalance your nutrients, but be patient. Depending on the size of your pores, plan to spend a minimum of one month changing this drawback.

Dry or flaky skin can be caused by a vitamin deficiency. By carefully balancing your nutrients you'll be able to change your body chemistry. Your skin will become naturally moist and radiant.

Drinking and Your Face

All my clients who eat too much carbohydrate retain water. And often the cause of a puffy or bloated face is too much wine, beer, or hard liquor. You can spot a big drinker by the following signs: a puffy face, a double chin and jowls, tiny broken blood vessels around the nose and cheeks. A big drinker will have other spots that are out of proportion, such as the stomach and back, but the face wll give a person's drinking habits away immediately.

I've had many clients who've written down all the food they ate, meticulously listing every bite, while somehow neglecting to write down what they drank.

Jack couldn't understand why he wasn't losing weight. I took one look at him and I could see from the puffiness that he'd been drinking too much. He had bags under his eyes and his double chin was just as pronounced as when he'd started the program. We discussed exactly what Jack had been eating and drinking. He admitted that at the end of the day he *had* to have a glass of wine to relax. "I used to drink martinis but now I'm only drinking wine. I even bought the 'lite' stuff."

Well, folks, the "lite" stuff just isn't light enough. You may be able to cut your daily bread out and cut down someplace else and lose a few pounds but your face won't reflect a healthy, radiant glow until you change your bad habits.

It's too easy to let yourself go wild when you drink. If you can handle one four-ounce glass of wine or one ounce of hard liquor a day, then you'll be able to have it on my program. If you don't drink or you want to get off alcohol, don't have even one glass of wine. Be honest with yourself. Drinking is one of the most difficult habits to change. It's social, it's comforting to some people, it's a way of relaxing for others. There are a million ways to rationalize drinking. If you want to hit this spot, be a purist! Don't be a weekday dieter and a weekend partygoer. You can't be successful doing both.

Plastic Surgery and Diet

I work with several plastic surgeons who refer patients to me prior to having a face lift. Dr. Frank Kamer, a well-known Beverly Hills facial plastic surgeon, explains why.

"You have to divide the patients who are always overweight from those people who lose and gain weight. The person who's always overweight usually should not try to lose weight before surgery. They are and often will continue to be overweight. The people who go up and down in weight must lose weight and stabilize it before having a face lift. I tell them to lose five pounds more than they want to so they'll have a little leeway.

"The Spot Reducing Diet is nutritionally sound. You lose weight slowly and then you have time to stabilize. I like my patients to stabilize for a month before having surgery. If you get a face lift when you're fat and then six months later go on a diet and lose weight you probably will not look as good. A person with a thinner face will have a better result than someone with a heavier face."

For those of you contemplating a face lift, please take Dr. Kamer's expertise into consideration. If you really want to look and feel your best, spend at least one month on the maintenance program before having surgery.

Face Foods

You can mix up avocado facials and oatmeal packs but if you don't nourish your face from the inside, you won't see a glow on the outside.

Makeup is a mask. It's a way of camouflaging your sins to build up your self-confidence. In my experience, many of the most beautiful women, such as actress Katharine Ross, wear almost no makeup because they know how to nourish their skin from the inside out.

Katharine came to me to lose a small amount of weight but mainly to learn good nutrition. "I've seen a difference in my skin since I started to include more vegetables in my diet. I think they do make a difference," she says.

Looking good *naturally* is the key. To roll out of bed in the morning and *feel* that you look beautiful or handsome can be your best reward.

Bobby Colomby loved eating junk food when he came to me. I promised him that if he learned to like vegetables and incorporate them into his diet, his face would slim down. He believed me, and made a point of having everything on the Master Plan every day. Going through sugar withdrawal was unpleasant but with the help of a piece of partial skim milk cheese and a piece of fruit, or a tablespoon of specially prepared peanut butter and a piece of fruit, he got through the worst of it.

It gave me great satisfaction to watch Bobby's fantastic transformation from big and heavy to tall and slender. It was a remarkable transformation: in all, he lost 50 pounds.

"People look at me now," he says, "and they say, 'Bobby, I can't imagine you fat.' That's because everything changed. My skin, my hair, my eyes—I mean everything! I got healthy!"

The Hit the Spot Glow

It is a *glow*, not a shine. A shine can mean that one has oily skin, whereas skin that radiates good health emits a glowing aura. People will automatically turn and look at you. They will feel something positive in you whether they know you or are simply admiring you from afar.

I attribute the Hit the Spot glow to the magic in vegetables. Balancing your nutrients gives you a spot-free, balanced shape, but it is specifically one's daily intake of vegetables that gives you the healthy glow I'm talking about.

Clients who say they don't like vegetables and cut down on what they're supposed to eat may lose weight but they won't get a look of good health. Their faces invariably get the gaunt, caved-in look. The same applies to fruit. If you think you can get by with less than your three servings a day you can, but you won't have that special glow.

How you feel is going to show in your face. You can camouflage a multitude of late nights and cartons of junk food but as the years pass, the telltale signs are going to become more and more difficult to hide.

Use your brain. Prevent sagging, bagging, wrinkling skin by learning which foods make you look puffy and unattractive and avoid them. Remember which foods give you the glow, especially vegetables, and make sure you include them in your daily eating.

The more attractive you are, the more people will find you attractive. The face and neck are two spots that won't keep a secret. Take good care of them and they won't have to.

Bags Under Your Eyes

Your whole face can become puffy and you can get bags under your eyes from consuming too much carbohydrate. Too much salt in your diet can also contribute to bags under your eyes.

Rosalynn ("Lolly") Hart came to me to lose ten pounds. She got far more than a perfectly balanced figure and an increase in her energy level. She was able to change her most annoying spot, the bags under her eyes.

"I was thinking of having the bags under my eyes removed surgically," she says. "They looked puffy and bad two weeks out of every month. Now I have them maybe one or two days a month. I solved the problem without surgery. I rebalanced my body when I balanced my diet. While I was on the program I lost ten pounds but I didn't lose one ounce in my face. My color is better, I have more energy, and I don't have saddlebags."

The reason Lolly was so successful is that she followed the program totally and patiently. She cut her intake of salt; she didn't use it at the table or in cooking. She also cut down on her intake of carbohydrate. "If you do it in two weeks," she says, "it'll come back in two weeks if you stop. The changes I've made I want to maintain forever."

Chin Up—the Double Chin

The double chin goes right along with yoyoing. Going from deprivation to reward repeatedly causes you to lose the elasticity in your skin, and one of the most annoying, unattractive side effects is the double chin. One of the biggest offenders in this area is alcohol. While you're hitting this spot, try the chin-up exercise. It will also help tighten jowls. Sitting up straight, tilt your head back and reach your lower lip out and over your upper lip. Hold for the count of five and release. Repeat this five times every day. It will help tighten this spot.

Jowls

Jowls tell me that you've gone from deprivation to reward too many times.

Reshaping your face is going to be a slow process but I have had clients who have successfully eliminated their jowls. Think of it as a healing process. If you slowly, patiently allow your jowls to disappear, they will do just that. And when I say slowly, I mean slowly.

It takes years of yoyoing to develop jowls, so plan to spend a minimum of two months losing them. You have to be patient, and when they've finally disappeared, be especially careful not to go back to your old eating habits. If you do, you'll have jowls as fast as you can eat a load of carbohydrate.

Eliminating jowls with diet is much more reasonable and probably longer lasting than doing it with plastic surgery. Facial exercises can help tighten up your jowls but exercise alone won't make a noticeable difference; diet will.

Wreath Around the Neck

A wreath around the neck and face is a prominent layer of fat circling the head. This is especially true for both men and women who drink too much or who eat too much carbohydrate.

I had a client whose husband is a movie personality. She asked me what he was doing to cause the wreath around his face. "In his last movie," she confided, "he looked like a squirrel with his winter supply of nuts stored in his cheeks—and it wasn't a comedy." His hobby was collecting vintage wine and every time anything happened, good or bad, it was time to open another bottle. He also loved dessert.

His wife said that at the first mention of a food program he became enraged. What could she do? He was about to start a new movie and was mourning the fact that his face and neck were fat. Even though he was losing his handsome leading-man looks he still wouldn't go on a diet because he was athletically active and was in good shape every place else.

I told her that it was wine and desserts that were giving him the wreath. The only way she could help him, I suggested, was by enlisting his help in her endeavor to hit her own spots. She was losing her midriff bulge and saddlebags.

She went home and told him that she couldn't drink for two months and would he help her by curtailing his drinking. He agreed because he really wanted her to lose weight. They made a bet that he could really stop for two weeks. In that short time away from the wine and high-carbohydrate desserts he saw the wreath around his face and neck shrinking. He became so enthusiastic about the change that he decided to stay on the program until he started shooting his film. By the time the cameras started rolling his wreath was gone and his face looked younger.

Aging and Your Neck

The neck is one of the spots that can give your age away fastest. You can take wonderful care of your face, but if you repeatedly lose weight *too fast*, the creases around your neck will betray even the best face lift. To prevent sagging skin around the neck lose weight slowly.

To tone a wrinkled neck, hit the spot for a minimum of one month. If you're patient you will be able to improve this hard-to-hit spot. A little exercise in conjunction with the program will help speed the improvement along.

Hair

Too much carbohydrate for the amount of protein and fat in your diet will make your hair dull, dry, and lifeless. And I'm not talking about hair damaged by too much sun, too many permanents or bleaching sessions. You can damage your hair from bad eating habits as much as you can from improper care.

Rebalancing your nutrients will ultimately bring the fullness and luster back. You won't need special shampoo, heat treatments, or conditioners to give you healthy, shiny hair. It will become beautiful naturally.

If you're balding, don't expect the Spot Reducing Diet to make your hair grow. It won't. It will, however, help you keep what you have. Too much stress can cause a person to lose hair unnecessarily. Balancing your protein, fat, and carbohydrate will make you a more relaxed person.

6

SHOULDERS

When they're out of proportion, shoulders are one of the most difficult parts of the body to camouflage—especially on girls and women.

The ones who seem to have the biggest problem in this area are young ladies who think that eating a lot of protein and athletic stamina go hand in hand. They don't!

When your body is out of proportion it's because your diet is out of balance. And if you look as if you have the weight of the world on your shoulders, it's because you're eating too much protein for the carbohydrate and fat in your diet. You may not even be aware of how much protein you eat. A piece of cheese here, a few nuts there, a glass of milk and a lean hamburger patty. All loaded with protein.

Protein fat is hard fat. When it's concealed by clothes it appears to be muscle, but when it's bare, uncovered for everyone to see, it has a hard, swollen, bloated look.

Men generally want the broad-shouldered Sylvester Stallone look. But girls of any age know that muscular shoulders are anything but feminine. They're enough to make the beach your last resort.

If you have corpulent, chunky shoulders, the chances are you need to lose weight all over. So, for those of you who think shoulders are just the beginning, see Chapter 12, "Face to Feet."

The Overnight Sensation

Slimming solid shoulders to achieve a lean, angular look is going to require patience, perseverance and a purist approach. Reshaping your shoulders means reproportioning your body, and that's going to take from six to ten weeks, depending on how much reshaping there is to do. Daily exercise will help speed the process along, but *be patient.*

Spot reducing sounds like magic to a lot of people. And when your body rebalances, it looks like magic. The time between starting the program and seeing that magic can be pleasant and exciting, or frustrating and eternal, depending on your attitude.

It is not a close-your-eyes-and-suffer diet. Don't expect to suffer for two weeks, see a dramatic difference, and go back to your old eating habits.

Be prepared to lose weight, to watch the needle on the scale slowly creeping downward, while your shoulders seem to be staying the same. Then, you'll wake up one morning, put your clothes on and suddenly find that your shirt is two sizes too large. *When the dramatic change happens, it happens overnight.*

Jane, a fifteen-year-old client, can help me illustrate this point. When she came to me she confided, "I know I'm too big, but it wasn't till some of the kids started asking if I was gonna try out for the football team that I got upset, really upset. I pretended it didn't matter at school but when I went home I cried till I couldn't see anymore. My mother wanted me to come to you but I didn't want to. I didn't think anything could help me lose weight in my shoulders."

Jane's mother had been one of my clients. She'd never had a waistline to speak of and came to me for that reason. It took her two months to reproportion her body so that for the first time in her adult life she was wearing belts and clothing that accentuated her waist. She insisted that her daughter try the program.

We analyzed Jane's eating habits. She was a very dedicated and competitive tennis player. She played daily and fueled herself with foods that she thought were good for her—a hunk of last night's roast, a protein shake, or a big slab of cheese. The food was good; it was just more than she needed. It was turning a pretty young girl into a big, muscular two-by-four. She was too embarrassed to wear a sundress or bathing suit.

It took Jane nearly two months before the dramatic change happened. And when it finally did—it seemed like an eternity to the teenager—it happened literally overnight. And not only were her shoulders lean and beautifully proportioned but so was the rest of her. Jane learned what had made her too big, she learned the meaning of good nutrition and how to balance her nutrients. Now she's an even better athlete because she's not carrying so much weight around. She can move faster, both on and off the court.

There is nothing more alluring than a woman with beautiful shoulders wearing an evening gown. Diana, Princess of Wales, nearly caused a riot when she wore a black strapless evening gown to celebrate her engagement to Prince Charles. Photographers went berserk and a new fashion trend swept the Continent.

If you need long-term inspiration, find a fashion photograph featuring Princess Diana or someone else whose bare shoulders will remind you what you *will* look like when *you've hit this spot*.

Born Broad

If you're one of those people who've always felt that your shoulders were too pronounced; if you were born with extremely broad shoulders and you'd like to shift the emphasis someplace else—there's hope!

If you aren't particularly overweight but would like to redistribute your weight, follow the Spot Reducing Diet over an eight-week period and your shape will show a dramatic change. You'll see improvement along the way but it takes weeks for your body to rebalance itself.

A perfectly proportioned body means eating protein, carbohydrate, and a small amount of fat, often hidden in other foods. Cheese, for example, is loaded with fat. Melt it and watch the pool of oil that forms. When you're eating protein you're usually getting an ample amount of fat.

Let's say that you've shaped your shoulders and you're still not satisfied with the way you're built. As far as you're concerned your shoulders are still too prominent. Okay, do the next best thing—learn to love them. Buy clothes that accentuate the parts of the body you want to emphasize. When you eat the proper balance, you feel centered, and when you feel centered you achieve a sense of harmony with your whole body. If you believe you look good you will transmit that positive feeling to others.

Ah, Men!

Men like their shoulders to appear broad and muscular. They've been raised to believe that macho means Superman, Christopher Reeve, and Burt Reynolds. The message in a lifetime of movies, television, and advertisements is that *real men* have broad shoulders. Whether real men have broad or narrow shoulders is irrelevant to me, but I've learned that it's a very sensitive spot with my male clients.

If you need to lose weight all over but don't want to trim your shoulders, exercise. Build your shoulders up while you're slimming down.

Now, if you just want to let nature take its course, you'll be pleased to discover that as your body slims down, as your shoulders lose weight, so will the other parts of your anatomy. When you've hit all the spots you're interested in trimming, you'll notice that your shoulders, even though they're smaller, will still appear broad in relation to the rest of your body. What you lose in weight you gain in good health and good proportions.

Fixing the Flab

Many of you have spent years building your shoulders up with weights, sports activities, and just plain work. What happens when you slow down; when muscle starts turning flabby? Is there hope? Yes!

As one gets older the skin has less elasticity. It becomes increasingly difficult to tighten flabby areas. After working with numerous clients, I discovered that if they ate a balanced diet and exercised moderately, their flabby skin and flabby shoulders began tightening right up. See Ron Fletcher's Whole-Body Toner Exercise, p. 217.

7

ARMS

Arms will become large and unattractive from too much carbohydrate. Too much fruit, too much wine, or too many sweets on a daily basis will give you that soft, gloppy, hanging kind of flesh.

This is not to be confused with big shoulders. Shoulders get a padded look from too much protein.

When Arms Hang Like Tired Wings

When I was 45 and ready to resume my career as a nutritionist, I decided that it was time to get myself in shape. *Slowly* I went from 170 down to 130 and in the process I lost a tremendous amount of weight in my arms—so much weight that I looked as if I'd sprouted little wings. I was so embarrassed by the loose flesh hanging down that even during a heat wave I wore long sleeves. I had not yet made the correlation between what one eats and the spots that are affected.

Then one day a former client called to make an appointment. "I've gained weight, Hermien," she said anxiously. "Only this time, not in my hips. It's my arms—I can't get my coat on. My arms are so huge they won't go through the sleeves!"

She came in and we discussed what she'd been eating. She was definitely out of proportion from the waist up and especially in her arms. It seemed that since losing weight the first time, she and her husband had moved to a beautiful new house in the country with its own apple orchard.

"I've been so careful," the woman told me. "I don't buy sweets and I never eat fat. I've been really good."

She was confused and so was I. I told her to write down everything she ate during the next week. There had to be a reason she'd gained 20 pounds in six months.

When I looked at her food cards, the cause became clear. Without even realizing it she'd been eating eight to ten large apples a day. I told her to cut down to three small servings of different fruits a day and we'd see what happened. It took about a month for her arms to shrink back to normal.

Perhaps, I thought, I could trim my flabby wings by cutting down my intake of fruit—I'd been eating six or seven servings of fruit a day. I cut down to three small servings a day and exercised. *This spot requires exercise along with a balanced diet.* I've watched people exercise strenuously and still manage to tighten the loose flesh only slightly.

It took me three months of carefully balancing my protein, fat, and carbohydrate, plus daily exercise similar to the one about to be described, to tighten this spot. And today, years later, I still have slim arms. They're not flabby and I'm not embarrassed to wear short sleeves.

The Circles Exercise

Standing tall, extend your arms straight out at your sides. With fingers pointing toward the ceiling—arms always straight—circle 20 times to the back and then 20 times to the front. If 20 times is too much at first, start with ten and build up.

Seeing the Change

Since every body is different, I can't tell you exactly how quickly you will be able to slim your arms. I've had clients who have seen a change in one week and others who have had to wait as long as a month. A lot depends on what you've done in the past. If you've been a pretty disciplined person rather than someone who repeatedly goes from deprivation to reward—arms are one spot especially affected by yoyoing—your arms will probably respond more quickly.

Older women get wrinkled, flabby arms after menopause because of the drop in their estrogen, and a lack of exercise. It will take an older person of either sex longer to lose weight and tighten this spot than a younger individual with more elastic skin. As in my case, patience and perseverance will result in slim, tight arms.

8

BREASTS

If I could tell women what to eat to make their breasts larger I'd be a billionaire sitting on the boards of both *Cosmopolitan* and *Playgirl*. Unfortunately, however, the breast is a very tricky spot. It is an area that changes very slowly—it may take as long as two months to see a really noticeable change. That goes for building up a flat bosom as well as reducing a very full one.

Small Breasts

In my experience, women who have small breasts in relation to the rest of their body are the ones who have repeatedly gone from deprivation to reward. They have gone to extremes, sometimes to the edge of starvation. They step on the scale and, having lost weight, they breathe a victorious sigh. "I need a reward," they tell themselves and off they go on a binge. And a binge usually means rich foods or sweets. The result may be a pear-shaped figure, one in which the top is much smaller proportionately than the bottom.

Most people believe that the less you eat, the faster you'll lose weight and the sooner you'll look better. Ironically, it doesn't work that way. When you lose weight too quickly you experience the fad dieter's pattern. Fat disappears from the face, the neck and the chest and by the time you reach the waistline it's as if someone's placed you in the deep freeze. The shape-changing process slows to almost a halt. Remember, it took time to set your shape and it's going to take time to reshape it.

Lolly Hart came to me to lose a very few pounds—ten, to be exact. Her primary objective was to reproportion her figure. "On previous diets," she explained, "I would lose maybe four or five pounds and it always appeared that I had lost weight from the waist up. My bust would look smaller. The top part of me looked smaller. My face looked drawn and haggard. My top looking smaller made my bottom look larger, so I would say, 'It doesn't matter if I lose five pounds!' So I would gain the five pounds back and everybody would tell me I looked healthier because my face looked better. And I appeared to have a larger bust. Now, after three months on the Spot Reducing Diet I've lost twice as much weight, my bust looks larger and my face looks just fine. My friends have commented that my bust looks bigger. To me it looks bigger too. That *could* be because I lost weight in the right places and therefore it appears larger; I did not lose any weight in my bust. The weight came off my hips, my stomach, my rear, and saddlebags. It was an amazing phenomenon."

Hello, Dolly!

We are still a nation with a sweater-girl mentality. Dolly Parton's huge bosom may be the extreme, but it nevertheless epitomizes womanhood to many people, so it's only natural that when you go on a diet you don't want your breasts to shrink. You want to lose weight where you want to—to hit your spot without compromising your femininity.

If you're concerned about maintaining your breast size or its proportion to the rest of your body, be sure to eat your daily allotment of dairy products. When you begin to lose weight, you will lose some of the fat inside the breast tissue, not the breast tissue itself. From my experience, having your daily allowance of fruits, vegetables, and dairy products is the key to saving your bustline from deflating and just hanging there.

If you're small-busted and want to enlarge this spot, adhere to the Master Plan precisely and substitute on the menus where necessary so that you will have dairy products every day:

1 oz. of cheese—see Cheese Exchange List, p. 56
⅓ cup lowfat plain yogurt

⅓ cup lowfat cottage cheese
½ cup vitamin A- and D-fortified nonfat milk

Never binge on fatty foods like chocolate, ice cream, or cheese and then try to undo the damage by starving yourself. It won't work! The breast is one of the most difficult spots on the body to change.

The women who *really* want to enlarge their breasts and are motivated to follow the Spot Reducing Diet with a purist's vengeance are eventually successful. The ones who either cheat or just take liberties with the program see very little change.

Every body is different, so it's impossible to give you a specific timetable. I had one client who was boyishly flat-chested and bottom-heavy. She had 25 pounds to lose from the waist down. Her goal: slim hips and a noticeable bustline. She followed the Master Plan even when she went on a vacation. She never binged and never went out on a limb. Weeks, then months, passed and although she'd lost the weight—her hips were down—she continued to hit this spot. It took six months for her body to redistribute her weight. Her bosom had finally gone up one whole bra size. And since her body was now perfectly proportioned, her bustline looked even larger. As the diaphragm goes down, one will look even bigger-busted.

You must be patient if you are going to see a dramatic change in this spot. Plan to spend months, not weeks, to reproportion your body and enlarge your breasts. It can be done!

Breast Reduction

Reducing a very full bosom is as difficult as trying to enlarge it. It's one of the slowest spots on the body to change. Again, be prepared to follow the program for weeks, maybe even months, before seeing a dramatic difference.

When a person is large-busted, the first spot to go down will be the back, the part that hangs over the bra. Then slowly, as the body loses weight and begins to reproportion itself, the area around the breast and down the back will slim, and the bust will look better. It must be done slowly or you'll lose the elasticity around the breast and have two flat pancakes.

Attitude has so much to do with successfully changing this spot. Most women who've come to me wanting to reduce their breasts have been convinced that they couldn't, so were scripted for failure from the onset. You must believe that you will be successful—and believing, you must not veer from the program until you've achieved your goal.

The clients who have reduced their breasts have combined my balanced nutritional program with exercise, as exercise alone will not reduce this spot. It is the combination of diet and exercise that allows the fat to leave the breast tissue slowly while the pectoral muscles are strengthened, thus pulling the breast up. The older you are the more difficult it is to lose weight without losing the elasticity in your breasts. Here is a simple exercise you can do at home each day. Start slowly with 15 and build the number up to 50 a day.

Breast-Lift Exercise

Stand approximately two and a half feet from the wall with your feet slightly apart (a wooden or uncarpeted floor works best). With your back and legs straight, extend your arms straight in front of you, with your palms touching the wall, and turn your fingers to face each other. Using your arms—elbows bending out wide—press your forehead to the wall. Keep your back and legs straight. Return to the starting position and begin again. These are standing push-ups and you'll find them very uplifting.

From my experience, the keys to breast reduction are:

1. Follow the Spot Reducing Diet *exactly*. Have three cups of vegetables *every day*. Eat a variety of vegetables. Also, be sure you're getting the correct amount of protein every day. Use your food scale.
2. Never binge. When you've achieved your goal you will be able to eat anything you can control.
3. Cut dairy products to a minimum. Where the menu tells you to have ⅔ cup of lowfat cottage cheese for lunch, substitute something from the Protein Exchange List, p. 55—turkey breast, tuna, shrimp, etc. Where it calls for ⅓ cup lowfat plain yogurt or lowfat cottage cheese as a snack, substitute a nondairy ounce of protein such as specially prepared peanut butter. Have only one ounce of cheese—see p. 56—*twice a week*. If you have to have milk, make sure it's vitamin A- and D-fortified nonfat milk. And never more than ½ cup.
4. Exercise your pectoral muscles every day. Even if it's for only five minutes, it's still worth while.

9

THE BACK

Eating and drinking too many carbohydrates relative to the protein and fat in your diet will give you a fat back. It's easy to see yourself coming but you can't always see yourself going, so it's easy to have pounds creep onto your back without even realizing it. When this happens to a great extent your back can have the appearance of an overstuffed laundry bag.

The back is another of the spots on the body that change *slowly*. When you hit the spots on your back—there are several of them—you may go along for a month before you notice a dramatic change. I have client after client who needs great tenacity and patience from one week to the next until *overnight* a shirt or brassiere is at least one whole size too large.

In the history of fashion no one has ever been able to design a blouse or shirt that can camouflage this ugly spot. Usually if a person has a fat back he'll have a big stomach and a big diaphragm as well.

It took me about six weeks to see a noticeable change. And then when it finally happened, I went down one brassiere size—and not in the cup, but around the back. The longer I continued to balance my nutrients, the more fat melted away, until I became a smaller person all over. My body slowly reproportioned itself. I went down two brassiere sizes—from a size 38 to a size 34. And overall I went from a size 20 down to a size 4. As my body shrank, so did my desire for huge amounts of fattening carbohydrates. Twenty-one years later I still wear a size 4 and love every thin, shapely minute of it.

Dowager's Hump

Dowager's hump is a big chunk of fat at the base of the neck that usually occurs after menopause. It's especially unattractive because it shows above a dress. But, like the other spots on one's back, it will disappear when one's intake of carbohydrate is balanced correctly with all the other nutrients.

Upper Hip Bumps

Traveling down the back to the spot just past the waistline and bordering the upper hip, one finds bulges caused primarily by alcohol.

One may have a small waist with a big handful of flesh on either side. I would say that three-fourths of my male clients have this problem. Most of them are big carbohydrate eaters and drinkers. And once again, by following the Spot Reducing Diet one can make these ugly, fleshy handles melt away.

The Lower Back

If the lower back is your problem see the discussion of posteriors in Chapter 11. Bulges in this area are caused by eating too much fat relative to the protein and carbohydrate in your diet.

The Huge Back

When Bill came to me he looked like a camel when he sat down. His back resembled an inflated cushion. This 45-year-old man looked bloated and had shortness of breath, with a small behind and thin legs. He was a man who never sat down to a meal. He lived alone and whatever was there he ate; he never planned a meal. Instead he sailed through his local supermarket picking up whatever struck his fancy. And in Bill's case it was always food high in carbohydrate, such as cookies, sweet rolls, candy, Cokes, bananas, crackers, cereal, honey, and jelly.

Whenever I'd say "vegetables" he'd point at his food card and say, "See, my corn! What're you talking about?" There's nothing wrong with corn unless you eat a whole can of it in one sitting. Bill ate nothing in moderation and the proof was that his back was as fat as his front. He also rewarded himself with several liqueurs after dinner every night.

This man was obese from eating so much carbohydrate. It took him six months to lose weight and reshape his body. Now he can wear a sports shirt without popping the buttons or looking as if he has an inner tube underneath. He stands taller and looks more attractive from both the front and the back.

It's easy to spot a woman with a huge back because her bra makes an indentation, accentuating the loose flesh hanging over it. The flesh actually hangs over the brassiere and even when it's covered with clothing this spot still bulges.

Remember, the back changes slowly; give yourself at least three weeks to hit this spot—and no cheating—before expecting to see a noticeable change. It will happen for you, just as it happened for me, if you're patient.

10

THE STOMACH AND WAISTLINE

When it's flat you love it and when it sticks out you try to hide it. You use every trick in the book from muscle control, control-top panty hose, girdles, plastic sweat wraps, jeans that make you walk like a wooden soldier, muumuus and caftans, or you just accept it and let it all hang over your belt.

The stomach (a word I am of course using in the sense of "abdomen") is one of those areas you can try to camouflage. You can try to fool others but when it comes right down to the buff, when it's between you and romance or you and your full-length mirror, size and shape are no secret.

What Caused Your Midriff to Bulge?

It's the little things, bites of carbohydrate here and there, plus a glass of juice or a drink that add up to a big stomach. Many of my clients don't realize which foods and beverages fall into the carbohydrate category. While they're hitting this spot they discover that it was the jam they put on their toast or the sugar-coated cereal with raisins and the waffles saturated in syrup that gave them more than a burst of energy for breakfast.

As you work on the midriff, all of your spots will shrink to their proper proportions. If you have an enormous stomach, plan to spend six weeks to two months flattening it. If you have only a tiny paunch, it's possible to bring it down in two weeks.

Actress Barbara Rush came to me because she was having a problem flattening her stomach. She was only a few pounds overweight but the excess poundage had all centered in her middle. Exercise and pounds-off diets could solve the problem temporarily but now she wanted to hit that spot permanently. The first step was to analyze her eating habits.

Life-style plays a major role in the way you gain weight, the way you will lose it, and the ways in which you can keep it off forever. Barbara was a social eater. Her calendar was booked solidly with brunches, lunches, and dinner parties. Parties for which the food was prepared by master chefs and gourmet cooks. Special gatherings at which the host and hostess feel deeply wounded if you refuse "their" fettuccine Alfredo or homemade bread. Saying "No, thank you, I'm on a diet" is generally followed by a round of "Which one?" and "Oh, come on, you can start your *new* diet tomorrow." In Hollywood it seems that everyone, with the possible exception of Orson Welles, is always on a diet.

Knowing which foods fall into the three categories is going to give you the ability to make the right choices for yourself. Every body responds differently to food and drink. Just as Barbara Rush discovered, if you listen to what your body's telling you, you will know which foods to stay away from and which ones to eat often. While she was hitting her spot, Barbara traded rolls and crackers for raw vegetables, and wine for Perrier water. Her stomach flattened to a smooth plane. Now she will always be able to maintain her perfectly proportioned figure. On the Maintenance Program, as you will discover, you can have your fettuccine Alfredo and wine, too.

Weight Distribution

If you don't really want to lose weight but your stomach is a little too noticeable, you can tone it down by rebalancing your nutrients. A small paunch will redistribute itself evenly throughout your body.

Joy Philbin came to me to lose her saddlebags. In the process she learned enough about spots to help her talk-show-host husband, Regis, rebalance his stomach without even realizing it.

"Regis just said to me the other day, 'That diet really works.' He didn't even realize that I was cutting him down on so many little things, like bacon in the morning. He loves fat too. He lost four pounds this week because I made him strawberry cloud for dessert instead of something fattening. I cut him down to diet margarine and I started scooping his bagels. I've been giving him the very thinly sliced rye bread instead of the regular, larger slices. And when we were on the tennis court the other day I said, 'Regis, my God, your stomach is flat!' "

Drinking and Your Stomach

Protein has four calories per gram, fat nine, carbohydrate four, and alcoholic beverages seven. Alcohol has more bounce to the ounce because it has more calories than you have with regular carbohydrate. Alcohol and fat will make you fat the fastest. And with alcohol, the higher the proof, the more calories per ounce.

One Scotch and soda contains about 150 calories. One glass of chablis contains about 85 calories and one 12-ounce beer about 160 calories. Have a few drinks and you won't need a calculator to figure out why your stomach sticks out.

You may also be suffering from water retention. Bloating is usually a result of consuming too much carbohydrate. Correct the imbalance in your diet and eliminate bloating.

Suzanne Somers used to enjoy a glass of champagne after her nightclub act in Las Vegas. "I do find that a glass of champagne is heavenly but after two weeks of just one glass a night I find a little bulge right here," she said pointing to her stomach.

Many of my male clients who have a paunchy stomach from drinking say, "Hermien, I won't give up drinking. I enjoy drinking! It relaxes me. Besides, I don't really drink all *that* much . . . never more than a bottle of wine in an evening."

"Then keep your spare tire!" I tell them. "You can't have a flat stomach unless you give up drinking for a few weeks. You can have one glass of wine with dinner and if you lose weight, fine. If you don't, that stops too until your stomach is down."

The ones who take my advice end up with a flat stomach, which makes them look taller and in all cases years younger. I don't know what it is about a spare tire but it always makes a young man look old and an old man look aged and heart-attack-prone. It adds years to a woman's appearance, too, but somehow it doesn't seem as dramatic. That might be because women wear girdles and slimming devices that can hide a multitude of sins.

The Magical One-Pound Drop

The *one-pound drop*, as I call it, is that magical moment when you have lost your paunch and along with it ten years. This is especially dramatic with men. At what point this occurs is totally individual. For some people it's five pounds and for others it's 50 pounds. The end result, though, is always the same.

Imagine yourself without your paunch. Visualize yourself with a flat, smooth stomach. It may be difficult at first, but keep imagining. Keep concentrating on the *new* you. *Put your imagination to work for you.* Movie stars do it before every film. They take a good look at the way they are. They imagine what they would look like if they went before the cameras today and what they *will* look like when they really step in front of them in three weeks. Knowing how you want to, and in some cases *have* to, look will help you achieve your goals.

Premenstrual Paunch

One excuse I hear repeated so often it makes my head ring is, "But, Hermien, it was just before I had my period. I always crave sugar before my period. I can't help myself."

You *can* help yourself. If you succumb to a monthly sugar craving you will never make it through sugar withdrawal, and the chances are you will never achieve a flat stomach on a permanent basis.

Bloating, or water retention, is a natural premenstrual side effect. But if you overeat carbohydrate, you'll make yourself even more bloated. Natural diuretics such as asparagus, alfalfa sprouts, tea, coffee, leafy green vegetables, and watermelon will help to minimize bloating.

Combining a lowfat cheese wedge and an orange, having half a frozen banana with specially prepared peanut butter or one cup of unsweetened strawberries or $\frac{1}{2}$ cup of peach slices will help satisfy your sweet tooth while allowing you to continue to hit your spot. The longer you are away from sugar the less you will crave it. You will actually find that a piece of fruit can be as satisfying as a piece of cake.

The Waistline

Your waistline does not have to spread along with the years. The reason this spot seems to expand with age can be subtle. It can mean eating a few crackers here, drinking a few glasses of wine there, a few beers and handfuls of pretzels after work or fruit juice and sugar cookies after school. Even children get thick through the waist from overeating carbohydrates.

Some people are so big all over that they don't have what you could actually call a waistline. Those individuals will discover that as they hit their other spots their waistlines will shrink to their proper proportions. It may take as long as two months before you see a dramatic difference in this spot, but I guarantee, if you do everything you're supposed to, you will have a waistline when you're finished.

One of my greatest thrills as a nutritionist is watching men and women who can't remember having a waistline develop one. It's exciting to watch women who have always camouflaged their thick midriffs with big shirts or bulky sweaters wearing streamlined dresses accentuated with a belt.

Men come in boasting when they can move their belt over one more notch. They practically jump up and down when they lose enough weight around their middle to buy a belt the next size smaller.

Five to Ten Pounds to Lose

Some people are not really overweight, but their bodies are out of proportion. They don't have a waistline to speak of, rather they are straight up and down. Barbara Martin is a perfect example of what I call a person with a boxy or rectangular look.

Barbara, a young airline hostess, was not fat, she was figureless. Her back and arms were fleshy with carbohydrate fat and her body was straight up and down instead of curving in at the waist. She was young, in her mid-twenties, but she was soft instead of firm. She could hide her unattractive spots by wearing a jacket, but when it came to wearing belts or clothes that accentuated her waistline, she couldn't do it. She wouldn't be caught dead in a bathing suit. When Barbara first came to me she said that she'd heard that I specialized in spot reducing but that she was absolutely certain that she could never lose weight in her waist. "I've never had a waistline," she said emphatically, "and I don't think there's anything I can do to get one!"

"This is the hardest kind of reducing," I told her. "It takes so long because your body doesn't have much weight to lose, rather, it has to redistribute your weight. And that's a slow process. Don't expect to see a noticeable change for at least a month." *You must go very slowly if your body is going to have a chance to reproportion itself.*

In Barbara's case she had to plan ahead if she was going to be successful. When she was air-hostessing she was used to eating whatever the passengers did. This means foods high in carbohydrate, such as crackers, Jell-O, and pretzels. When she was on the ground she liked to drink beer. I told her she'd have to switch to mineral water until she was ready for maintenance.

While she was hitting this spot, Barbara carried small cans of tuna packed in water, Laughing Cow Green Label cheese wedges, a jar of specially prepared peanut butter, and Baggies with vegetables with her. She knew that she would always be able to meet her daily requirements while traveling.

When the body redistributes weight it's very important that you follow the program *exactly*. Never have a glass of beer or a bowl of pudding and a sugar cookie because it's there. It took Barbara two months to lose five pounds and to redistribute her weight. For the first time in her adult life she had a thin, curvaceous waistline. She was wearing belts, bikinis and tight sweaters without jackets. "Hermien," she said happily, "I don't know how to thank you. You did it. I still can't believe it!" She pivoted around to show me how tiny her waist was. "It's a miracle," she went on.

"Wait a minute, Barbara. Let's get this straight. *I* didn't do it, you did. It wasn't a miracle. It was balancing your nutrients and being a purist about it for two months. You did it and if you don't do everything I tell you to do on maintenance, you'll undo it."

"Oh, Hermien, don't worry!" she said as she flew out the door.

Even though Barbara knew what caused her to be thick through the waist she didn't really believe me. She rationalized going back to her old eating and drinking habits and her waistline expanded accordingly.

Two months later she was back in my office. "Look at me," she wailed. "I'm straight up and down again. I even tried another diet and I lost weight every place but my waist. You've got to help me."

The reason I've recounted this story for you in detail is that Barbara is like many of my clients. She preferred to believe that her waistline had become smaller as a result of a miracle and that I was the one responsible. I may be the one responsible for giving you the tools with which to spot-reduce but you are the one who must make your own miracle—especially when redistributing weight.

Once again Barbara spent two months hitting her spot. The second time around she knew that *she* was the one who earned her small waistline and that she was the one responsible for keeping it the way she wanted it *for her lifetime*. She had lost seven pounds and seemingly all of it from her waistline. Since that spot was the one most out of proportion it was the only one that had obviously changed.

To insure her continuing success Barbara went out and bought a whole wardrobe of belts. She gave away all the clothes she used to camouflage her thick waistline and she pasted a list of the worst waistline offenders on her refrigerator as a permanent reminder.

Hitting This Spot Without Losing Weight

If you want to streamline your waist without losing weight follow the Master Plan *exactly*, but add one teaspoon of butter or fat to your daily requirements. Depending on how much out of proportion you are, it may take you a few weeks or as long as two months to reproportion your body.

If you find that you're losing weight, add a little more protein or fat to your diet. It is the balance of nutrients that will cause your body to reproportion itself and since it was excess carbohydrate that made you thick through the waist, be sure that you never exceed your daily allotment. And again, be patient! You may have to go along for weeks before seeing a noticeable change.

Exercise and Your Waistline

Julie Carmen was a young professional dancer in New York City before coming to Hollywood to become a very successful film and television actress. "I used to think that I was destined to have a high waist and a puffy belly," she says. "But when I found out that all the dancing and exercise in the world wasn't going to make my waist smaller—when I found out that it was overeating bread and pasta—I changed my eating habits. I balanced my protein, fat, and carbohydrate. As I lost weight my body reproportioned itself. My thighs went down, my stomach went down, and my waistline became much smaller. Now that I know what caused my spots I'm careful to balance my nutrients. I know, for example, if I overeat bread I'll get thick through the waist."

It doesn't matter how much you exercise; if you really want to have a slim and trim waist, you must eat a carefully balanced diet in conjunction with being physically active.

Older people tend to get thick through the midriff because they are less active than they used to be. Age should not be a consideration here. Exercise is an appetite deterrent. While you're on the program and long afterward, it will help you to maintain your shape. See Ron Fletcher's exercise guide in Chapter 20.

A Waist of Drink

I have many clients, especially men, who come to me with their stomachs hanging over their belts. They don't have a waistline because they drink too many alcoholic beverages. They get that loose, gloppy carbohydrate fat that hangs over their belts and obliterates any notion of a waistline.

The same unattractive look can result when a person drinks too many soft drinks or too much fruit juice. I have clients who come in boasting, "I drink a couple of quarts of fresh orange juice every day. I'm into healthy food." As I've noted in the Master Plan, a glass of orange juice is comparable to eating three oranges. If you drink a quart of orange juice you are probably getting a dozen oranges without even realizing it. Oranges are loaded with natural sugar. Apples are too. Fruit in general is loaded with natural sugar; if you consume too much, the body stores the excess as fat—around your waistline.

Keeping It Small

Once you've trimmed your waistline, you should keep it that way. Dr. Richard Mettel, a Beverly Hills gynecologist, lost 30 pounds on the Spot Reducing Diet in three and a half months. When he was finished he looked ten years younger because of his slim new waistline.

Dr. Mettel was so thrilled with his new shape that he went out and bought several very expensive suits. He loved carbohydrate but he loved his well-proportioned body even more. Every time he was tempted to eat or drink more than his daily maintenance allotment he would think about his new suits and how fantastic he looked and felt wearing them. Dr. Mettel explains, "I know when I go off the maintenance program I start to get heavy around the middle. The weight goes right back where it was before. What makes a dieter successful is changing his eating habits. I have a small can of tuna packed in water and some vegetables every afternoon and when I get home from work I like to have a bowl of the vegetable soup. It's delicious hot or cold."

As Dr. Mettel says, "The Spot Reducing Diet has been the only diet that I've been able to adopt as an enjoyable way of life. I lost weight and I've kept it off. I'm not even scared to get on the scale anymore!"

11

POSTERIOR, HIPS, THIGHS, SADDLEBAGS, AND CALVES

When one or more spots on the lower part of your body are out of proportion, it is because you have been consuming too much fat for the amount of protein and carbohydrate in your diet. If you have repeatedly yoyoed from deprivation to reward, losing weight and gaining, losing and gaining, you will probably be much smaller on top than you are on the bottom.

I have dozens of clients with big hips or saddlebags or thick calves who say, "But, Hermien, I don't eat much fat at all. I don't use much butter, I use diet mayonnaise, I even use 'light' salad dressing." They are emphatic because they know exactly how much obvious fat and oil they use but they have no idea how much *hidden* or *invisible fat* they're getting. Many of these people are fat addicts without even knowing it.

Hidden fat is as insidious as sugar. You may find yourself making certain food choices because of the fat content. There are fat fish and lean fish: salmon and whitefish are much higher in oil than shrimp or sea bass. Avocados, nuts, and cheese are loaded with hidden oil. TV dinners and chunky canned soups can be very high in fat. Always read the label.

Dr. Lesley Z. Blumberg, a gynecologist, came to me to streamline her hips and in the process learned just how much hidden or invisible oil she was getting. "I tended not to notice the hidden fat in certain cuts of beef or certain types of fish," she says. "Everybody said all types of fish are low-calorie—well, some of them are as fattening as or more so than beef. So after starting the program I began to have an awareness of invisible as well as the visible fats. And if I intend to keep my hips down I will have to continue to be aware of my intake of fat and oil."

Fat is essential to our daily diet; there are three essential fatty acids that we neither make nor store. Also, fat-soluble vitamins like A, D, E, and K must be in fat to be soluble. Fat insulates and lubricates the skin and cushions the organs. It stores fuel and has great satiety value because it leaves the stomach after protein and carbohydrate. It keeps you feeling full longer. You need fat—but only *in moderation*.

Posterior

I have clients who say, "Look how thin I am, Hermien!" and when they turn around they have a regular shelf in the back.

There are certain ethnic groups who seem to have their weight concentrated in their posteriors. Many of these people have given up changing their bottom-heavy shape because they believe they inherited it and there is nothing they can do to change it. That's just not true.

You may have inherited a body type or a tendency from your family, but your big behind was caused by overeating fat. In fact, you may have been overeating fat since you were a child. Your whole family may suffer from this imbalance but that doesn't mean that you can't lose weight and reproportion yourself.

Greek and Italian cooking is loaded with olive oil; soul food is heavy with oil and frying fats; even so-called health-food fanciers get this look from eating too many avocados, nuts, and seeds, and too much safflower and sesame oil. Too much of any good thing will give you great big spots.

Linda Lane came to me to trim her posterior and legs. "I thought because I was a writer," she says, "that I had a big behind from too many years of sitting at the typewriter. This may sound silly but I didn't really think I ate much fat. A friend told me about spot reducing, and after years of dieting that never hit the spots I wanted to lose I went to Hermien. She took my food history and there it was. Without knowing it I was a fat addict. I was big on cheese, chicken legs, salmon, and baked potatoes stuffed with sour cream. I didn't really believe I could lose weight in my backside and thighs but after years of being bottom-heavy in a town with lots of perfect size eights, I gave it a try. It took about three weeks before I saw a dramatic change. When I started I wore an eight on top and a twelve or fourteen on the bottom. When I finished two months later, I wore a size eight on both the top and the bottom. I was a new person, psychologically. I felt competitive. I had more energy and a much greater sense of self. The more attractive I became, the more my social life expanded."

Hips

Suzanne Somers completely changed her shape when she hit this spot. She recalls, "My hips used to be very high. When I stopped eating fats this went away and suddenly my hips lowered and looked the way I'd always wanted them to. I had amazing visual results." Every time you want to eat something that contains a lot of fat, just remember that if you eat it you will wear it!

Jean Kasem used to have a pear shape. "I went on the Spot Reducing Diet and within a week Casey and I saw a noticeable difference on my hips and thighs alone. And now that I'm on maintenance I'm very careful about what I eat. It's not worth cheating. It's not worth feeling sick or feeling guilty because you ate three pieces of fried chicken and you know your hips will be an inch bigger."

Protein Fat

Often people feel that protein is low in calories. That is not necessarily true. Much protein also contains hidden fat. Cheese, for example, is high in fat, so eating big hunks of it will give you big hips and thighs.

Thighs and Saddlebags

The majority of celebrities I've worked with have come to me to trim their hips and thighs. When they have dieted in the past they've lost weight too fast. When you lose weight fast you don't lose in the right spots.

Sandy Duncan was my first client at Ron Fletcher's. She came to me because she wanted to increase her energy level and trim her saddlebags. She started the program with two pounds to lose and redistribute. She went week after week without seeing the dramatic change I promised her would occur when she balanced her nutrients. Sometimes when you have very little weight to lose it takes longer than if your whole body is losing all over.

Sandy would call me and in a frustrated voice say, "Hermien, I still can't get into my jeans." I told her to stick with the program and she would, *soon*. Then one morning, two months into the program, she called and said, "Hermien, last night I couldn't pull my jeans up and this morning I can't keep them up!" She was ecstatic.

There is an epilogue to Sandy's story. She moved to a new house that had a beautiful avocado tree. She forgot avocados are rich in oil, so before she knew it she had saddlebags again. She stopped eating an avocado a day and this time in only two weeks her saddlebags were gone.

The Dramatic Change

If you have that dimpled, cottage-cheesy type of fat that forms along the outer thigh and is called cellulite, you are eating too much fat *and carbohydrate* for the amount of protein in your diet.

Unlike a fat back or thick calves, this ugly, dimpled fat comes from combination foods, like chocolate candy, rich dessert mousses, heavy puddings made with cream, pound cake, or very rich ice cream. You may not even be overweight but still have cellulite.

It is possible that you keep your caloric intake low so that you aren't really overweight but you'd rather not be seen in a bathing suit. The solution to eliminating this unattractive spot is rebalancing your protein, fat, and carbohydrate. Follow the Master Plan and you will watch the loose, dimpled flesh melt down and tighten up. Eating properly is preventive medicine.

Men

People don't usually think that men get fat from the posterior down, but I have a large percentage of male clients with large behinds and big thighs. One reason is that they live alone and when they eat out, which they often do, they eat fried potatoes and fried meat and lots of gooey salad dressing. Usually they don't drink much alcohol but those who do go in for Piña Coladas or Kaluha and cream. They are usually people who keep chips, cookies, and chocolate candy in their homes. They're junk-food junkies who would rather take a cold shower than cook vegetables for themselves. The first thing they tell me is that they like corn and peas and that's it when it comes to vegetables. The other ones are foreign to them unless they happen to be French fried zucchini or onion rings. Some are gourmets who love rich sauces. They all love butter and oil. They are all fat addicts.

In order to hit their spots these men have to change their eating habits along with balancing their protein, fat, and carbohydrate. They have to learn to like vegetables and fruit. They have to re-educate their tastebuds.

Thighs

Joy Philbin is a perfect example of someone who had a minor figure flaw and was able to change it by changing her balance of nutrients. "I have a small frame," she says, "and if I'm five pounds overweight, it shows. Regis and I had gone on a cruise and I was a good eight pounds overweight, but I thought, 'No problem—I'll go home and it will fall off me.' My thighs had been getting heavier and heavier as I got older and I thought it was something I was going to have to live with and I reconciled myself to it. But when I gained the eight pounds on the cruise I didn't want to put on a bathing suit. So after about a month and a half of dieting at home and there was an improvement, I saw Victoria McMahon and was so impressed by the transformation in her legs I couldn't believe it. Her figure was perfect. At first I thought it was silly to go to a nutritionist to drop eight pounds. I could certainly do it myself, but nothing happened. So I went to Hermien. I went on the Spot Reducing Diet and I didn't notice any real change until six or seven weeks later when I walked down the stairs in my tennis skirt and I happened to catch my reflection in a mirror. It was just like that—one and a half inches off each of my thighs, and I hadn't lost a significant amount of weight. If you eat fats and you eat a lot of meat and fried food it's going to go right to the thighs."

As Joy mentioned, her friend Victoria McMahon came to me and trimmed her saddlebags. Victoria recalls, "When I first met Ed he was on a diet and I went on it with him. I lost weight then but I never lost the saddlebags. And I was probably thinner than I am now. I had been given stories of, 'Well, there's someone in your family who is heavy and you have this body form from them. I was told that that was why I could never get rid of them. I even went to someone who pounded them out. It's only since doing the Spot Reducing Diet that I've kept them from coming back and it's been three years."

Victoria lost 22 pounds and in the process completely eliminated her saddlebags. She wouldn't wear pants or jeans until she hit her spot. Ed McMahon likes the Spot Reducing Diet because it gives him increased energy.

Your New Look

Cyndie Freeman went from being a bottom-heavy 30-year-old to, as she says, "a long, lean lady."

"I was contemplating thigh-reduction surgery when I started the program. I'd been on every diet in the world—Weight Watchers, liquid protein, I'd gotten shots, I'd done everything you can do to lose weight and nothing gave me a well-proportioned shape. I was so desperate to lose weight that I cut way down on my protein until I was protein-deficient. I got stuck at 133 pounds and I was eating 500 calories a day and my chemistry was shutting down. Hermien insisted that if I would follow her balanced program I would feel healthier and lose in the right spots. I didn't believe her but I'd tried everything short of surgery, so I ate everything she told me to. It was so much more food than I was used to.

"It took three months for my body chemistry to get back into working order but when I was finished, for the first time I had a small tush and thin legs. Now I find that I can date and I approach any social situation with flexibility. The world now thinks I'm thin. Also, right after I started the program I went through a sudden divorce. Normally I'd have gained thirty pounds from hand-to-mouth disease but because of the balance of the Spot Reducing Diet I got through the whole mess and lost weight."

Calves

Heavy calves usually start developing early in one's life. They are another spot that takes time to change. If you are slim in other places but wish to hit this spot, plan to follow the Master Plan with a vengeance for a minimum of four to six weeks before seeing a dramatic change. It will happen if you have the patience to wait until your calves are much thinner overnight.

If you are bottom-heavy *and* have thick calves, you will be pleased to discover that as your posterior melts away your calves will slim down right along with them.

Exercise

It is absolutely possible to trim your posterior, hips, thighs, saddlebags, and calves using the Spot Reducing Diet without an exercise program, but it takes longer. I recommend exercising for one hour four times a week. It will make your spots disappear faster.

See Ron Fletcher's exercise guide in Chapter 20.

12

FACE TO FEET

When a person is big and solid all over, it's from eating too much protein for the amounts of carbohydrate and fat in his or her diet. Clients with this shape usually say, "It takes me longer to lose weight than other people because I'm so solid." They believe this because they've tried to lose weight in the past and have experienced the typical dieter's syndrome: their faces get thin, even gaunt; they lose weight in the chest, and by the time they get down to the waistline they've given up.

Most of my face-to-feet clients are young and athletic, although, every once in a while, I'll have a middle-aged man or woman who has so consistently overeaten protein—huge amounts of cheese, 16-ounce steaks, pounds of nuts, and quarts of whole milk—that their shapes have grown to Amazonian proportions. They are chunky or hefty.

Recently Sue, a 20-year-old English girl, approached me at a wedding reception and said that she would very much like to lose weight all over but she didn't think she could. "I'm a nanny," she explained. "I take care of two little girls. I cook their meals and I have to make sweets when they have friends round for tea."

I explained that her problem wasn't sweets as much as it was protein. "Yes," Sue acknowledged, "I've always been a big protein eater—cheese, yogurt, eggs. . . . Yes, I guess I eat a lot of protein."

"You know," I told her, "you'd be a knockout if you'd lose 30 pounds." She had an absolutely beautiful face and a lilting personality but she was so tall and solid that most of the young men at the reception were swarming around Monica, her thin friend.

As a test I gave Sue the Spot Reducing Diet. "Because you're so tall," I told her, "have ten ounces of protein a day instead of nine. And watch it! Measure everything, and if you find yourself getting ravenous, eat a bowl of the vegetable soup or some vegetables. If you follow the right balance you'll see your excess weight melt off you evenly. But be patient, Sue. Give it a minimum of six weeks."

Two months later Sue called and asked if she could stop by. "I have something to show you," she explained.

When I opened the door I was awestruck. She'd lost 20 pounds. Her face was full and radiant and she hadn't lost any weight in her bustline. The 20 pounds had simply melted off her whole body *evenly.* Sue did a 360-degree turn to show me how well proportioned her body was. She was a smaller person.

"I just did what you told me to do, Hermien. I stopped tasting the children's food. I stopped eating loads of meat and yogurt. I cut down to four eggs a week and here I am," she said enthusiastically. She winked and added, "I even did a few things on my day off that we won't talk about."

Sue still had another ten pounds to trim but she had changed her eating habits and she was so pleased with her new shape and the compliments she was getting that I could tell she would stay on the program until she reached her ideal weight.

In order to hit this overall big spot one has to balance his food completely. The people who fall into this category are always the hungriest of my clients, because they must reset their appestats before they can become successful dieters.

It takes 20 minutes for your appestat to get the message that you've had enough to eat, so if you cram yourself with food you'll eat more than the person who seems to take forever, the person who gets the message that he's full in time to stop. Remember: it takes only 50 extra calories a meal, or 150 extra calories a day, to make you 15 pounds heavier in one year. For example, three and a half ounces of broiled salmon can contain as much as 700 calories. If you eat a big salmon steak, you could be getting as many as 1500 calories. The recommended daily allowance for an adequate diet is set at 2000 calories by the Food and Nutrition Board, National Academy of Sciences, National Research Council. So if you're used to eating large servings of protein throughout the day you're probably getting thousands of calories more than your body can use and the excess is being stored from head to foot in the form of solid or hard fat.

The reason my face-to-feet clients seem to be the hungriest when they limit their food intake is that they've been ignoring their "full" signal for so long that it's completely out of whack. If this is your trouble, eat sitting down and eat slowly. Both will help you reset your appestat. It's important to understand that *it's not terrible to feel hungry*. If you are afraid to feel hungry, then you must be committed to eating low-calorie foods after you've hit your spot; otherwise you'll put all the weight back on again. In any event, you have to lower your intake of food if you're going to reset your appestat.

It takes about three weeks to conquer the insatiable urge to eat. A typical face-to-feet meal might begin with a shrimp cocktail, a 16-ounce steak, a baked potato stuffed with sour cream, broccoli covered with cheese sauce, whole milk, and caramel custard. You may think that sounds like a wonderful meal but there's too much protein for the amounts of carbohydrate and fat. It is this very imbalance that makes you hefty all over.

Many of my clients have no idea how much they eat until they have to write everything down. If this is your spot it's *especially* important to write down everything you eat and drink every day. Before bed, add everything up to make sure you've met your daily hit-the-spot requirements *and* that you haven't gone over your protein allowance.

One of the main reasons Sue successfully hit this spot was that she measured everything she ate and wrote down everything she ate and drank for the first month. Now she can look at a slice of turkey breast and decide whether it's four ounces or six. She developed food sense.

In my experience, being too big and solid all over affects more men than women. I have male clients who eat from 15 to 20 ounces of protein a day and say, "I don't eat a lot of protein." They genuinely don't think they do because their appestats are set so high they *think* their bodies need that much. They don't!

One way to appease yourself during a ravenous period is to eat lots of vegetables. Like many of my clients, you may regard vege-

tables as something better to look at than to eat. And like those same clients after giving vegetables a real chance, you may find that they're more delicious than most of the foods you now crave.

Bobby Colomby lost 50 pounds on the Spot Reducing Diet and in the process learned to appreciate the *essence* of food, especially of vegetables. "I didn't eat vegetables before I went on the program," he admits. "I used to get so much sugar and salt in the food I ate I couldn't really taste anything. Now I can taste everything, including the hidden ingredients. Vegetables are fantastic. When Hermien says they have magic, I believe her!"

Make a button bag (see p. 159), raw vegetables in a zip-lock Baggie, if you know you have hand-to-mouth disease and you can't stand feeling hungry. It will help you reset your appestat, lose weight, and change your eating habits.

You're probably under the impression that if you're hungry, protein is the best thing to eat. It *is* good for you, but too much protein will make you fat.

13

THE BIGGEST OFFENDERS FOR EACH BODY SPOT

Face and Neck

BIGGEST OFFENDERS:

wine, beer and alcohol, carbohydrates: puffiness, bad color, broken blood vessels in cheeks. Neck will get thick.

highly fatted things, rich meats and cream sauces, heavy cream, rich desserts: give you tiny bumps beneath the eyes like whiteheads that, unlike pimples, don't go away and must be professionally removed. This condition occurs over a period of time with people who have lots of fat in their diet.

candy	An excess of:
cookies	bread
crackers	cakes
honey	matzos
ham	pancakes
jelly	pasta
molasses	pies
regular chewing gum	popcorn
sherbet	pretzels
sugar	waffles

All chips are a double-edged sword—they contain both too much carbohydrate and too much fat.

Too much fruit: Fruit is only as good as the vitamins and minerals it provides. If you eat more than your three fruits a day, generally speaking, it becomes like ordinary sugar and your face will get round and your neck may get fat or thick.

Arms, Back, Waistline, and Stomach

BIGGEST OFFENDERS:

alcoholic beverages—wine, beer, hard liquor, liqueurs
bread
cake
candy
canned fruit
cereal—sugared
chewing gum—regular
Coffeemate
cornstarch—cornstarch-thickened sauces
cookies—those high in sugar, such as Oreos and granola bars, are especially bad for waistline (stay away from all cookies while on the Master Plan).
crackers
dried fruit
English muffins
flour—flour-thickened sauces
fruit—too much
fruit juice
gravy
hard candy
honey
jam
Jell-O
jelly
ketchup
matzos
molasses
nectars, such as peach or pear
pancakes
pasta
pies
popcorn

Popsicles
Postum
pretzels
pudding
raisins
sauces thickened with cornstarch, flour, or arrowroot
sherbet
soft drinks
sugar
sugared cereals
syrup
tapioca pudding
tonic water—regular
tortillas
waffles

Posterior, Hips, Thighs, Saddlebags, and Calves

BIGGEST OFFENDERS:

anything au gratin
avocado
bacon
baked goods high in butter or shortening—stay away from
beef—marbled or highly fatted
breaded anything, if fat or oil is added
butter
caviar
cheese
chicken legs
all chips
chocolate
cream
cream and cheese sauces
cream soups made with whole milk or cream
creamed cottage cheese
croissants
cocoa
coconut
dark meat of poultry (legs, thighs, wings)

Hit the Spot!

dips
doughnuts
duck and goose
eggs—too many
fatty fish
fatty meat—highly marbled meat, lunch meat, smoked meat, dried meat
fish roe
fried food—all
hors d'oeuvres
ice cream
imitation ice cream
lunch meats
margarine—too much
mayonnaise—too much, or any type of mayonnaise dressing
meat soups—not skimmed of fat
mousses
nuts
nut butters—particularly if some of the fat is not removed
olives
olive oil, vegetable oil, corn oil—any kind of oil
pastries
pâté
piccata—done in butter
pork products
pot and farmer cheese—read the label to see if they have added cream
potato chips
potato salad or cole slaw made with a lot of mayonnaise and/or cream
poultry skin
pureed vegetables—usually loaded with cream and butter
quiche
ribs
salad dressing—all regular
sausage
sautéed foods
seeds
sour cream
sweet rolls
TV dinners—most
veal—fatty cuts such as veal breast

wieners
whole milk and whole-milk cheese
yogurt—except lowfat or nonfat

Face to Feet and Shoulders

BIGGEST OFFENDERS:

Too much protein:
meat
fish
poultry
nuts
Highly fatted proteins can also cause heavy behinds, thighs, knees, and big calves:
duck
highly fatted cheeses such as blue, Cheddar, Brie, etc.
fatty meat such as veal breast, short ribs, fatty brisket and pork ribs
salmon
butterfish
Too many dairy products:
cheese
regular milk
yogurt
Teenagers: You need calcium, but it's best to cut way down on your milk intake. Ask your doctor about using a calcium supplement while you're on the program. That will enable you to lose weight more effectively while still getting all your nutrients. Lowfat cottage cheese and lowfat plain yogurt are also excellent sources of calcium.

HIT THE SPOT RECIPES

14

LOW-CALORIE GOURMET DISHES

Whether you're making dinner for one or 21, the recipes in this chapter will help you create mouth-watering, sumptuous-looking taste treats that are truly low in calories. Many so-called low-calorie recipes are really *lower*-calorie recipes; they've had one or two of the most fattening ingredients omitted but they're still too fattening for someone who wants to change his shape. Stay away from lower-calorie dinner dishes until you've hit the spot and are ready for Maintenance.

In this chapter you will discover how you can entertain lavishly without adding fuel to your friends' spots. *Do not tell your guests they're eating a diet dish.* Suzanne Somers was a gourmet French cook before becoming a gourmet spot-reducing cook. She says, "It's wonderful to do an absolutely scrumptious, delicious meal where no one has any idea that they're eating a meal that is, for lack of a better word, a diet dinner. No one has any idea and they don't feel as though they've missed anything. They haven't! They've had a nutritious, delicious meal that won't put an ounce on anybody!"

Those of you who wish to share your low-calorie secrets will have fun with dishes such as turkey baked in a bag, paella, and strawberry cloud. The whole family will enjoy making as well as eating many of the recipes. Remember, you don't have to be on a diet to benefit from the Spot Reducing Diet's nutritional balance.

If you don't like, can't get, or can't afford something on the daily program, you've come to the right place. Flip through the recipes that are of comparable value—a dinner for a dinner, a vegetable for a vegetable—and substitute one recipe for another. You're allowed beef or lamb only twice a week. Don't go over your limit. Watch the substitutions and be careful not to make dishes that are labeled Maintenance. Many of the celebrity menus are for Maintenance.

Many of my clients have grown so fond of cooking with dry vermouth or a nonstick coating such as Pam instead of butter or oil, or keeping a pot of vegetable soup or ratatouille in the refrigerator to take the edge off hunger, that they have happily incorporated the low-calorie spot-reducing methods and recipes into their daily lives.

Just because your mother made it fattening, that doesn't mean you have to. Victoria McMahon told me that her mother was always a wonderful cook who put butter or sauce on squash, broccoli, green beans—everything. "I steamed broccoli for her and now she thinks it's wonderful. Now she cooks that way. I went over to my cousin's house and she not only was putting butter on the squash, she was putting sugar on it. This is a great example of a thin person with large hips. I asked her why she was cooking with so much butter and she said, 'I've cooked like this forever.' She didn't realize that by changing the way she was preparing vegetables she could make her figure better balanced."

Drinking

While you're hitting the spot you are allowed only one four-ounce glass of dry white wine in exchange for your day's bread allotment. Suzanne Somers serves her guests wine as well as ice water. She believes that the presentation is as important as what you're serving.

"I keep ice water on the table in beautiful crystal glasses. I put a lemon slice and a sprig of fresh mint in it. When you pour the water, it almost has the quality of nectar; it's very subtle. And once your guests get used to drinking it, I've noticed that everyone starts pushing his wine glass away. They drink the water because it's so refreshing."

Joy and Regis Philbin are constantly entertaining and being entertained. Joy notes that in Hollywood things have changed. "You always have to have Perrier or some kind of mineral water on hand. Many people don't drink hard liquor at all. I find that wine and

Perrier are the two things you *must* have in the house when you entertain now."

The trend in and out of Hollywood is to look and feel your best. The celebrities who have contributed menus to this chapter are some of the happiest, healthiest, most perfectly proportioned people I know. Follow their lead as you hit the spot.

Enjoy!

How to Brown or Braise with Vermouth

1. Take 2 T. very dry vermouth, add onions and/or garlic, and cook until onions are translucent.
2. Dip meat, veal, or chicken, in ice water for 1 minute.
3. Let drain, but don't pat dry.
4. Turn heat up under vermouth and onions as far as it can go. (You don't see the vermouth, it just coats the skillet.) The very cold meat put into the very hot skillet with vermouth sears or browns the food. It browns quickly, so watch it. Don't let it burn.
5. Take off the fire and add broth or wine, and bake or simmer.

Fish

Take 2 T. very dry vermouth and cook onions and/or garlic. Wash fish, cover with lemon juice, let drain but don't pat dry. Put into the freezer for 2 minutes. Then follow directions 4 and 5 above.

Joy Philbin's Ladies' Luncheon for Six

snow peas with tuna and anchovy dip
soy chicken (see p. 154)
asparagus vinaigrette
brown rice with water chestnuts
chilled fresh fruit
white wine spritzers
coffee or Sanka

SNOW PEAS WITH TUNA AND ANCHOVY DIP

½ cup low-calorie mayonnaise
1 8-oz. container plain lowfat yogurt

1 6½-oz. can tuna, water packed, drained
1 2-oz. can anchovies, drained
2 T. lemon juice
½ t. paprika

    In a food processor or blender, blend all ingredients until smooth. Trim 1½ pounds snow peas and drop into boiling water for 1 to 2 minutes. Drain and rinse under cold water. Arrange around dip on large, round platter. Sprinkle dip with 1 T. capers, if desired.

ASPARAGUS WITH LOW-CALORIE VINAIGRETTE DRESSING

2 pounds fresh asparagus, steamed
2 t. Dijon mustard
⅓ cup chicken broth
1 whole garlic clove, peeled and mashed
½ t. minced fresh parsley
2 leaves fresh minced basil or ½ t. dry
1 T. wine vinegar
1 T. lemon juice
½ t. freshly ground black pepper

    Combine all ingredients except asparagus in tightly lidded jar and shake well. Refrigerate until flavors blend. Before using, remove garlic and shake again. Makes ½ cup. Pour over chilled, steamed asparagus and garnish with chopped egg, if desired.

FRESH FRUIT FLAVORED WITH LEMON JUICE

1 fresh pineapple
½ medium honeydew melon
3 nectarines
½ pint strawberries
2 T. lemon juice

    Cut pineapple and melon into cubes and nectarines into wedges. Leave strawberries whole if they are not too large. Combine the fruit in a bowl and toss with lemon juice. Chill and serve in fruit cups.

Katharine Ross's Beach Menu

marinated chicken breasts
pasta salad—only if you are on Maintenance
fresh fruit

MARINATED CHICKEN BREASTS

Marinade:
½ cup lemon juice
¼ cup corn oil
½ cup chopped onion
1 t. tarragon
Tabasco, to taste

Marinate chicken at *least* ½ hour or as long as overnight. Broil or barbecue chicken about 30 minutes. Baste while cooking. Drain and chill.

PASTA SALAD

rigatoni noodles
baby shrimp, cooked
broccoli
vinaigrette dressing

Cook rigatoni noodles as per directions on box but do not add salt to cooking water. Rinse in cold water and drain. Cut a broccoli head in small flowerets and steam until crisp, then plunge in cold water and drain. Mix noodles, baby shrimp, and broccoli together in a bowl and add vinaigrette. Serve cold.

VINAIGRETTE DRESSING (MAINTENANCE ONLY)

¾ cup salad oil
2 T. lemon juice
2 T. white wine vinegar
black pepper, ground
crushed garlic
1 t. dry mustard
fresh chopped basil

Combine all ingredients in a blender or in a tightly covered jar.

ALTERNATE DRESSING FOR PASTA SALAD

Serves 6

2 T. Weight Watchers or Light n' Lively mayonnaise.
Dilute with one, two, or all of the following ingredients:
mustard—regular or Dijon
lemon juice
water
vinegar

Suzanne Somers's and Alan Hamel's Dinner for Ten

shredded crudité
bouillabaisse
mango

SHREDDED CRUDITÉ

romaine lettuce
zucchini
carrots
beets
celery

Finely shred zucchini, carrots, beets, and celery separately in a food processor. Place a mound of each shredded vegetable on romaine lettuce leaves on individual plates. Serve vinaigrette dressing on the side.

BOUILLABAISSE

2 lbs. assorted shellfish: lobster, crab, scallops
1 can clams (use broth)
1 lb. assorted fish fillets, such as halibut, red snapper, sole
2 T. dry vermouth
1 cup chopped onion
1 lb. can Italian peeled tomatoes
2 cloves garlic, minced

⅛ t. fennel seed
½ t. basil
½ t. thyme
¼ t. ground allspice
½ cup chopped parsley
1 cup dry white wine
¼ t. saffron (optional)
1 bay leaf
1 T. lemon rind, grated
2 t. oregano
¼ t. black pepper

Sauté onions and garlic, add all ingredients and bring to a boil. Simmer 20 minutes covered and 20 minutes uncovered. Place in a large soup tureen.

If you are on Maintenance, try Suzanne's idea of decorating her bouillabaisse with a flower made of filo dough. Place 3 or 4 sheets of buttered filo dough over the bouillabaisse and twist into the shape of a flower. Place in oven till dough is cooked.

MANGO

Cut mango in half and remove the seed. Place mango on plate with piece of fresh lime and some mint leaves.

Jean and Casey Kasem's "Top 40" Family Dinner

Serves 6

Hit the Spot vegetable soup
baked potatoes with butter or diet margarine
scallops Hermien
Jean's fruit ambrosia
(for vegetarians: steamed vegetables)

HIT THE SPOT VEGETABLE SOUP

1 box frozen green beans or ¾ lb. fresh green beans
1 green pepper, sliced or chopped

½ large or 1 whole small cauliflower, cut into flowerets
6 stalks sliced celery
¼ cup chopped parsley or celery leaves
2–4 large yellow onions, sliced or chopped
1 16-oz. can peeled tomatoes
1 16-oz. can V8 juice
4 packages George Washington Golden Broth or M.B.T. chicken broth
2 T. thyme
1 package frozen whole baby okra (optional)

Mix all ingredients and simmer for 15 minutes.

NOTE: This recipe makes a large pot of soup that will keep for two weeks in the refrigerator.

SCALLOPS HERMIEN

1½ lbs. scallops
½ lb. medium to large cooked shrimp, shelled and deveined
3 T. dry vermouth
garlic powder, to taste
onion powder, to taste
dry mustard, to taste
thyme, to taste
pepper, to taste

Place shrimp and scallops in the freezer for 2 minutes. Remove and dip in vermouth. Season lightly with a combination of garlic powder, onion powder, thyme, dry mustard, and pepper. Place the seafood in a steamer that contains 3 T. vermouth as well as water. Steam for about 10 minutes or until the scallops are done. Serve with steamed vegetables.

JEAN'S FRUIT AMBROSIA

"I select as many kinds of fresh fruit as possible. Naturally, your choices will change according to the seasons. I cut them up, mix them all together and serve in either a tall champagne glass or a broad champagne glass. On top I add a dollop of plain lowfat yogurt. In the tall champagne glass, I layer the fruit with a dollop of lowfat yogurt."

Hit the Spot Recipes

For vegetarians:
"I use a fluted knife to give carrots, squash, etc., a pretty look before steaming them.
"Casey is a vegetarian and in order to get his 9 oz. of protein a day he may have all of the following:
    1 glass nonfat milk
    2 oz. partial skim milk cheese
    4 oz. plain lowfat yogurt
    1 T. specially prepared peanut butter
    1 serving lowfat cottage cheese
Occasionally he'll have a lobster."

A poolside snack for the whole family:
Frozen bananas with specially prepared peanut butter or apple slices sprinkled with cinnamon and served with thin slices of jack cheese. *Never peel the apple.*

Victoria and Ed McMahon's Dinner for Twelve

spinach salad
rack of lamb Dijon
steamed crisp green beans
strawberry cloud

DIET SPINACH SALAD

4 bunches fresh spinach
sliced fresh mushrooms
Baco Bits
chopped egg white
diet salad dressing

    When you think spinach has been washed sufficiently—wash it once more. Nothing is worse than sand in salad. Lay spinach abundantly onto plates, top with sliced mushrooms, and chill in refrigerator. Remove and add cold diet dressing sparingly. Sprinkle with Baco's (only if you're on Maintenance) and chopped egg white.

RACK OF LAMB DIJON

leg of lamb
Dijon mustard
red table wine
garlic buds
fresh ground black pepper

Wash leg of lamb and sprinkle with pepper. Pierce lamb and insert sliced garlic buds. Mark incisions with toothpicks so that garlic can be removed after cooking. Cover lamb evenly with Dijon mustard. Place parsley sprigs alongside lamb. Place in moderate oven (300°) and, using a meat thermometer, cook until done. Half an hour before lamb is finished, baste with red table wine. Remove lamb from oven and take out garlic buds. Wrap lamb in foil and keep hot. Let drippings settle in the freezer so the fat comes to the top. Skim off all fat. Slice lamb and serve with hot juice on the side. When buying your lamb, plan on 6 to 8 oz. of meat per person and remember that it will shrink. You may have gravy only when you're on Maintenance.

STEAMED CRISP GREEN BEANS

Place small amount of water in cooking pan—½ inch or less, depending on amount of fresh green beans to be cooked. Place one or more chicken bouillion cubes or packets of George Washington Golden Broth in water, then add beans. Steam 5 minutes or until done and remove while still crisp.

STRAWBERRY CLOUD

Serves 6

8 crushed ice cubes
2 cups frozen unsweetened strawberries (Kern's Fresh Frozen unsweetened, if you can get them)
2 egg whites
1 t. vanilla
dash of Sweet 'n Low

Crush the ice cubes; if you don't have an ice crusher, place them in a plastic bag and hit them with a rolling pin or a hammer. Place crushed ice in a food processor or blender and whirl. Add egg whites. While the food processor is running add strawberries, vanilla, and Sweet 'n Low. Stop machine occasionally to stir mixture. If it's too thick, add a small amount of water. Keep machine running until the mixture has become a light, frothy strawberry cloud. It tastes like ice cream. If you can drink it or it's icy, it hasn't been processed long enough. When it is finished it will be very smooth and you should eat it with a spoon.

To double the recipe, you will have to make a second batch, as one batch fills a food processor.

HIT THE SPOT FRENCH TOAST

Serves 1

2 slices very thin sliced whole wheat bread
1 egg
diet sweetener
cinnamon
½ t. vanilla
1 t. diet margarine or butter

Beat the egg and add a tablespoon of water. Add a dash of diet sweetener if you want, vanilla, and cinnamon. Place bread in egg mixture. Spray skillet with Pam or other nonstick coating and heat. Place bread in heated skillet. Brown one side, add 1 t. butter or diet margarine to the skillet and turn the bread over.

LOW-CALORIE SPINACH SOUFFLÉ

Serves 6

3 packages frozen chopped spinach
1 package frozen chopped onions or
   2 medium fresh onions, diced
8 oz. fresh mushrooms, sliced
4 egg whites, beaten until stiff
2 t. garlic powder
2 t. onion powder
2 t. dry mustard

mozzarella, American Lite Line, or Laughing Cow Green Label cheese wedges

Steam or boil spinach, onions, mushrooms, garlic powder, onion powder, and dry mustard in a small amount of water. Drain well and pour into a soufflé dish or casserole. Add beaten egg whites and mix well and quickly. Place slices of mozzarella, American Lite Line, or Laughing Cow Green Label cheese wedges on top of mixture. If you use Laughing Cow wedges on top, spread them out with a knife when they get hot and melt. Bake at 350° for 30 minutes.

HERMIEN'S LUSCIOUS *LOWER*-CALORIE SOUFFLÉ

You may have this only if you are on Maintenance!
6 whole eggs plus 4 whites
¼ cup nonfat milk
4 cups of shredded Lite Line Cheddar cheese
1 bunch green onions, sliced (use tops and part of green)

Beat the eggs until they are frothy—about 10 minutes. Spray soufflé dish with Pam or comparable diet nonstick coating and pour the eggs in. Add shredded cheese, nonfat milk, and sliced onions to the eggs, beat together. Place in a 300° oven and bake for 45 minutes to one hour.

NOTE: If it's high on the sides and low in the middle, it's not done yet. When it's ready it will be high and brown on the top.

Serve with steamed vegetables and fresh fruit. Artichokes go nicely with this delicious brunch dish. You may wish to serve very thin sliced toast with diet margarine or butter or English muffins. You know what you are allowed that day.

Lower-calorie means that the dish contains fewer calories than usual because one or more ingredients has been omitted from a more fattening recipe. The *Settlement Cookbook's* baked cheese soufflé calls for whole milk, bread crumbs, 4 tablespoons of butter, ¾ cup cheese, and only 4 eggs.

My souffle is lower in calories than its counterpart but it's still not a low-calorie dish. It is a recipe I recommend for clients on Maintenance because it's too easy to eat more than 1 oz. of cheese without realizing it.

NOTE: If you are watching your cholesterol, do *not* use this recipe.

TOMATO, MUSHROOM, AND ONION OMELET

Serves 1

2 eggs plus 1 extra white per person
1 T. nonfat milk
1 t. parsley, chopped
mushrooms, thinly sliced
tomatoes, thinly sliced
onions, thinly sliced
black pepper, to taste

Beat the eggs and milk, add parsley and pepper and pour into hot Teflon skillet which has been sprayed with nonstick coating.

When your omelet is nearly cooked, place the skillet under the broiler for 2 minutes, then add the fresh tomatoes, mushrooms, and onions. You may want to steam the mushrooms first. Place beneath the broiler for another few minutes, remove. To make a Spanish omelet, add chopped green pepper.

NOTE: Measure your vegetables before adding them to the omelet.

CHEF SALAD

Serves 8

chicken breasts, cut in strips (plan ½ per person)
cold roast beef, cut in strips (plan ⅛ to ¼ lb. per person)
½ lb. Swiss cheese, cut in strips—if you are on Maintenance
½ lb. American cheese, cut in strips—if you are on Maintenance
½ lb. jack cheese, cut in strips—if you are on Maintenance
every raw vegetable you can find, cut in flowerets, slices, or strips
1 lb. cooked bay shrimp
croutons—if you are on Maintenance
Baco Bits—if you are on Maintenance

Put each ingredient in a separate bowl and let your guests make their own individual chef salad. Make several kinds of dressing, such as thousand island, French, bleu cheese, and a diet dressing, and let your guests choose.

Because you didn't put dressing on the ingredients, save the leftovers and next day put them in a pot with 2 cans of chicken broth, which you have skimmed. Boil and puree it and you have a heavy vegetable soup. Add any herbs you like. Serve the salad with toasted English muffins, bagels, or hot French bread.

HIT THE SPOT COLE SLAW

Serves 4

½ small, fresh regular cabbage, shredded
½ small, fresh red cabbage, shredded
1 green pepper, chopped fine
1 small onion, chopped fine
1 bunch red radishes, slivered
2 carrots, slivered
¼ cup parsley, finely chopped
vinegar to taste
Sweet 'n Low, to taste (optional)
rosemary, to taste (optional)
tarragon, to taste (optional)
   Mix all together and chill.

SALADE NIÇOISE

Serves 1

romaine, Boston, or red leaf lettuce
2 or 3 oz. tuna packed in water (amount depends on
   your protein allowance)
2 egg whites, chopped
¼ cup green or red onions, chopped or thinly sliced
1 medium tomato, sliced
¼ cup green beans, steamed and chilled
parsley, chopped
   For the dressing see Hermien's handy dandy diet dressing.

TUNA SALAD

Serves 1

2 or 3 oz. tuna packed in water
¼ cup celery, chopped

green onions, chopped (optional)
1 t. Weight Watchers or Light n' Lively mayonnaise diluted with one or all of the following: lemon juice, mustard, vinegar, or water
curry powder or dill, to taste (optional)

Squeeze water out of tuna and weigh before adding the other ingredients. Don't rely on the weight stated on the label, as contents may weigh less when the water's been drained.

NOT ALLOWED: Tuna packed in oil. Even washing will not remove enough oil for you to effectively hit the spot.

MALIBU TUNA

Serves 4

1 13-oz. can tuna packed in water
4 chopped egg whites
¼ cup chopped celery
½ cup green onions (use ⅔ of the green onion), sliced
3 T. diet mayonnaise
3 T. vinegar (never rice vinegar)
2 T. mustard (Dijon or regular)
¼ t. curry powder, or more if you wish

Drain the water, add all ingredients and mix. (The easiest way to measure how much tuna you're getting is to weigh the number of ounces you have coming to you at dinner and then add the other ingredients.) Place tuna mixture on top of beefsteak tomato slices and grill under the broiler for 5 minutes or until brown. Count the mayonnaise as your fat for the day.

COLD HALIBUT SALAD

Serves 4

Sauce:
5 fresh tomatoes
1 medium onion, chopped
garlic powder
onion powder
Tabasco sauce
1 additional tomato, chopped
a drop of Liquid Smoke (optional)

Puree the 5 fresh tomatoes, garlic, and onion powder to taste, drop of Tabasco sauce, and Liquid Smoke. Add the chopped onion and additional tomato to sauce—it gives it character.

Fish:
1½ lbs. halibut fillets
lemon juice
2 T. dry vermouth
1 medium onion, chopped

Preheat oven to 350°. Wash fish, cover with lemon juice, place in freezer for 2 minutes, then sear in vermouth and chopped onions. Place in baking dish and cover with the above sauce. Bake for 45 minutes. Chill and serve, or serve hot.

MARINATED FISH FILLETS

Serves 4

1½ lbs. fish fillets

Marinade:
2 T. dry vermouth
¼ cup Worcestershire sauce
2 t. tarragon
2 t. mild soy sauce
1 medium onion, shredded
¼ t. pepper
1 bay leaf
1 t. garlic powder
1 drop Liquid Smoke (optional)

Combine marinade ingredients in a shallow dish. Add fish, cover and refrigerate for 4 hours or more. Turn fish occasionally to keep both sides moist. Remove from the marinade. Place on a broiler pan and broil 3 inches from the flame for 10 minutes or until the fish is done.

SPICY FISH FILLETS

Serves 4

1¼ lbs. red snapper or sea bass fillets
½ cup dry white wine

1 4-oz. can diced green chilis or 1 jar capers
1 small jar pimentos, chopped
2 medium tomatoes, diced
   Place fish in a baking dish, sprinkle green chilis or capers on the fish. Add tomatoes and wine. Place under the broiler for 12 minutes or until the fish is done. Remove from oven and sprinkle with pimento.

POACHED SNAPPER

Serves 4

1¼ lb. red snapper fillets
1 cup dry white wine
1 cup chicken consommé
1 T. lemon juice
1 t. dill
   Heat wine and consommé in a skillet, add fish, lemon juice and dill, cover and simmer for 10 minutes.

PAELLA

Serves 12

1 lb. crab, lobster, or scallops
1 8-oz. can clams in juice
1 lb. shrimp
1 can oysters, drained (optional)
2½ lbs. chicken breasts, boned and skinned
2 T. dry vermouth
¾ cup chicken stock
¾ cup to 1 cup dry white wine
2 cloves garlic, mashed
1 t. basil
1 lb. mushrooms, sliced
1 can Italian plum tomatoes
1 onion, sliced
1 cup uncooked brown rice or wild rice
1 T. paprika
½ t. saffron

¼ cup pimentos
1 15-oz. can artichoke hearts, drained

Heat oven to 350°. Sauté chicken and onion in vermouth and garlic. Combine all ingredients in a large casserole and bake for 1 hour. Add artichoke hearts for the last 10 minutes of baking.

HIT THE SPOT CHICKEN KIEV

Serves 6

6 chicken breasts, boned and skinned
1 oz. per serving lowfat mozzarella cheese or string cheese
2 T. parsley, chopped
2 t. garlic, chopped
black pepper
¼ cup cognac
1 cup chicken broth
3 T. very dry vermouth
toothpicks

Heat oven to 350°. Pound each chicken breast half with the flat side of a meat mallet to ¼ inch thickness. Sprinkle seasonings evenly over chicken pieces. Cover surfaces with grated cheese and roll up each half breast with cheese enclosed. Secure with a toothpick. Heat vermouth in a large frying pan and sauté chicken rolls until golden brown, about 8 minutes. Place in a shallow baking dish. To make sauce, add cognac and broth to drippings. Return to heat and heat to boiling, stirring constantly. Spoon over chicken. Cover; bake 30 minutes. Remove toothpicks before serving.

CURRIED CHICKEN

Serves 4

3 lbs. skinned chicken breasts, cut into serving pieces
2 medium onions, chopped
1 lb. mushrooms, thinly sliced
1 T. lemon juice
1 clove garlic, minced
1 T. curry powder
2 T. vermouth
1 T. Dijon mustard

½ t. onion powder
1 cup chicken broth or bouillon
⅛ t. thyme
⅛ t. pepper
½ t. ground ginger
2 firm green apples, cored and diced

In a large frying pan brown chicken pieces in vermouth; remove and place on a platter. In same pan sauté onions and mushrooms. Stir garlic and curry powder into onion-mushroom mixture. Add wine, broth, thyme, pepper, ginger, onion powder, and mustard. Stir and cook until mixture starts to simmer. Add chicken and simmer for 50 minutes or until done. Cook cored, diced apples in a small covered saucepan until soft. Add apples to chicken mixture; heat through but do not boil.

CHICKEN À LA FRAC

Serves 4

4 breasts of chicken, boned and skinned
6 T. lemon juice
2 cloves garlic, mashed
¼ cup chicken broth
black pepper, to taste
paprika, to taste

Pound chicken breasts with a mallet until thin. Marinate them in the lemon juice, garlic, pepper, and paprika for at least 1 hour. Simmer them quickly in the chicken broth, or you may sauté them in a frying pan coated with a nonstick coating such as Pam. They will cook very quickly.

POACHED CHICKEN WITH VEGETABLES

Serves 6

6 chicken breasts, skinned
2 carrots, cut in coin-size pieces
1 medium onion, sliced
1 clove garlic, minced
½ cup parsley, chopped

2 large stalks celery, chopped
1 bay leaf
½ t. thyme
2 cups chicken broth (skim off fat)
1 cup dry white wine

    Preheat oven to 350°. Place chicken breasts in a deep casserole or Dutch oven. Place all other ingredients on top of chicken breasts. Cover and bake for 45 minutes to 1 hour. Serve chicken with vegetables and broth.

SOY CHICKEN

Serves 4

3 lbs. chicken breasts, split and skinned
Green Label Kikkoman (mild) soy sauce
onions, chopped
mushrooms, sliced
garlic powder, to taste
onion powder, to taste
dry mustard, to taste
black pepper, to taste
dry white wine (optional)

    Heat oven to 350°. Dip chicken breasts in soy sauce and get them brown all over. Add garlic powder, onion powder, dry mustard, and pepper to each breast. Cover with chopped onions and loads of sliced fresh mushrooms. Cover with foil and bake for 45 minutes. Remove foil 5 minutes before removing from oven. If dry white wine is used, remove foil 10 minutes before taking out of oven.

TURKEY BREAST IN A BAG

Serves 4

turkey breast, skinned
mild soy sauce or Dijon mustard
onion powder, to taste
black pepper, to taste
garlic powder, to taste
curry powder, to taste

1 apple, sliced
1 onion (red if you can get it), sliced

Preheat oven to 375°. Cover breast with soy sauce or mustard, then sprinkle onion powder, garlic powder, pepper, and curry powder over it. Spray roasting pan with nonstick coating, place foil over it. Take a large brown grocery bag and place apple and onion slices inside, then place turkey breast on top of them. Fold opening of bag under and place in roasting pan. Bake for 2½ hours. (Don't worry, the bag won't catch on fire! Roasting the turkey in the bag will keep it moist.)

HAMBURGER
OR
ENCHILADA, TACO, OR TOSTADA STUFFING

Serves 4

1 lb. lean ground round or veal
½ t. pepper
1 T. cumin
2 T. chili powder
1 clove garlic, mashed
1 can tomatoes
1 T. garlic powder
1 T. onion powder
1 T. dry mustard
½ cup chopped onions

Mix all ingredients and simmer together for 1 hour if to be used for enchilada, taco, or tostada stuffing. If you are going to make a hamburger, omit the can of tomatoes, mix rest of ingredients and shape into patties; broil until done.

CHILI CON CARNE

Serves 6

2½ lbs. lean ground round or veal
1 cup red onions, chopped
1 qt. tomato juice
1½ cups canned tomatoes, mashed

2 T. chili powder
1 clove garlic, chopped fine or ½ t. garlic powder
¼ t. ground black pepper
1 4-oz. can diced green chilis (optional)
vermouth

Sauté onions in vermouth and set aside. Cook meat in a heavy saucepan until brown. Add onions, chili powder, garlic, tomatoes and tomato juice, cumin, and black pepper, and cook for 10 minutes. Add chilis and let simmer an additional 20 minutes.

SPICY LIVER

5 oz. calves liver or chicken livers per person
Hit the Spot hot tomato sauce (see p. 161)
2 T. dry vermouth
1 medium onion, chopped
½ green pepper, sliced
2 medium tomatoes, diced

Preheat oven to 350°. Sauté chopped onions in vermouth until brown. Dip liver in ice water for 1 minute, remove but don't pat dry. Turn skillet up as high as it will go and quickly sear or brown the liver. Place in a casserole or baking pan, cover with Hit the Spot hot tomato sauce, sautéed onions, ½ cup sliced green pepper and diced tomatoes. Bake for 45 minutes.

VEAL STEW

Serves 4

1½ lbs. very lean veal stew meat; cut into 1 inch cubes
2 T. dry vermouth
2 T. mild soy sauce
1 large onion, chopped
1 cup canned or fresh tomatoes
¼ t. black pepper
¼ cup chopped pimento
1 clove garlic, minced (optional)
1 t. rosemary
2 small carrots, sliced thin
½ t. grated lemon rind

⅓ cup celery, chopped
½ lb. fresh mushrooms, sliced
3 pieces fresh ginger cut in strips ¼ inch wide

Heat vermouth and soy sauce in a large frying pan. Sauté veal and onion until brown. Add tomatoes, pepper, garlic (if desired), rosemary, ginger, lemon rind. Cover and simmer for 45 minutes. Check occasionally and add water if needed. After 45 minutes, add carrots, green peppers, pimentos, celery, and mushrooms. Continue cooking for 30 minutes more or until veal is tender and vegetables are done. Add extra water if necessary. Garnish with lemon rind. Serve with brown or wild rice.

VEAL LOAF

Serves 4

2 lbs. very lean ground veal round or turkey breast that you have ground yourself
1 clove garlic, minced
1 T. Worcestershire sauce (or to taste)
1 large onion, finely diced
¼ cup parsley, chopped
½ cup red wine
1 T. mustard (Dijon or regular)
1 t. basil
black pepper to taste

Combine all ingredients in a loaf pan and bake at 350° for 45 minutes. Do not use the gravy.

VEAL SCALLOPINI

Serves 3

2 slices very thin sliced wheat toast, crumbed
¾ oz. Parmesan cheese
1 lb. veal scallopini (thinly sliced veal)
1 egg white, slightly beaten
2 T. vermouth
1 medium onion, diced
Hit the Spot ratatouille (see p. 159)

Mix bread crumbs with Parmesan cheese. Dip veal in egg white, then in bread crumb mixture. Brown in vermouth and diced onion. Place in a baking dish and cover with Hit the Spot ratatouille and bake at 350° for 30 minutes.

NOTE: If you prefer, leave veal in skillet and simmer with ½ cup chicken consommé, 1 T. lemon juice, and ½ cup dry white wine for 35 minutes.

BEVERLY HILLS GOULASH

Serves 6

1½ lbs. lean veal, turkey or chicken breast, ground
1½ t. paprika
1½ medium onions, chopped
⅛ t. dried marjoram
1 clove garlic, finely chopped
1 t. rosemary
1 t. thyme
1 t. basil
12 small white onions
1½ cups beef broth; you may use canned or cubes
½ cup dry white wine
1 small can of unsweetened tomatoes
2 T. finely chopped parsley
1 large or 2 medium potatoes, sliced
dry vermouth

Sauté onions and garlic in vermouth or Pam. Set sautéed onions and garlic aside and brown the ground veal, chicken or turkey breast. Pour fat off and add onions, garlic, and seasonings. Stir and add beef broth and wine. Add tomatoes and potatoes, cover and simmer for 40 minutes or until potatoes are soft.

BAKED POTATO SKINS

You may have one baked potato skin *free* each day. Buy the largest potatoes you can find—russets or Idaho. Scrub well, put fork holes in them and bake as you normally bake a potato, 1 hour at 400°. *Do not wrap or grease.* (I do 7 at once.) When they have baked and are still hot, slice and scoop the potato out, leaving the hard core next to the brown. Put all potato skins in the refrigerator. Place the insides in a bowl and mash for the rest of the family or freeze for later use.

Every day take out 2 halves or 1 large potato skin and place it in a 400° oven for 5 minutes or until hot and crunchy. You may choose to have your daily cheese allotment here. Place the cheese inside potato skin and melt in the oven. You may also enjoy the skin stuffed with tuna or chicken salad.

BUTTON BAG

Whenever you think you might need a snack or aren't going to get your allotment of vegetables during the day, make a button bag. Prepare any vegetable you can cut like a coin, such as carrots, celery, zucchini, cucumber, or make into flowerets, such as broccoli or cauliflower, and put in a Baggie. You can also cut string beans into thirds and you can have whole small mushrooms. These vegetable button bags can travel with you to the office, in the car, or on a plane.

HIT THE SPOT POTATO CHIPS

1 small potato per person

Wash thoroughly and cut into very thin slices. Do not peel. Spray a baking sheet with Pam or other nonstick coating and smear it with a paper towel or your hand. Place individual potato slices on the sheet and bake at 350° for 40 minutes or until brown and crisp. For best results, check them periodically, removing them as they become brown. Make sure they come out crisp or they'll become soggy quickly.

HIT THE SPOT RATATOUILLE

Serves 12

1 eggplant, peeled and cubed
6 zucchini, sliced
6 fresh tomatoes, cut up

1 large can Italian-style plum tomatoes
1 green pepper, chopped
2 large purple onions, chopped
loads of fresh mushrooms, whole or sliced
The following to taste:
  dry mustard
  garlic powder
  onion powder
  black pepper

Boil for 45 minutes. When cooked, sprinkle 1 T. Parmesan cheese over the whole pot. Do not put cheese on individual servings.

This is a versatile dish—good hot or cold. Fish or chicken can be baked in it. I boil shrimp and crab in it and serve it over rice. It will keep for 3 weeks in the refrigerator.

Another hint—put it in the blender and puree it and then serve it as a hot or cold soup. It makes a good snack or first course.

SPINACH WITH ONIONS

Serves 2

1 package frozen chopped spinach
1 medium onion, chopped
onion powder, to taste
garlic powder, to taste
dry mustard, to taste

Steam frozen chopped spinach, onion, onion powder, garlic powder, and dry mustard. The seasonings flavor the dish while it is steaming. Steam 10 minutes or until done.

STEAMED VEGETABLES

Select the vegetables you would like and steam them 4 to 5 minutes. You may add garlic powder, onion powder, curry powder, or dry mustard to the cooking water. When done you might like to sprinkle them with dry roasted onions, fresh chopped parsley, or chives—any herb or spice you choose. Steamed vegetables can be kept in the refrigerator for several days.

HERMIEN'S HANDY DANDY DIET DRESSING

1 6-oz. can tomato juice
2 t. Dijon mustard (more if you like)
1 t. lemon juice
2 t. or 1 T. capers
1 chopped egg white
garlic powder or fresh pressed garlic, to taste
black pepper, to taste
2 t. chopped pimento (optional)
 Mix well and chill.

HERMIEN'S HOT TOMATO SAUCE

1 medium onion, minced
3½ cups tomatoes, pureed in blender
2 cloves garlic (optional)
2 T. chili powder
½ t. ground cumin (optional)
¼ t. dried oregano

Sauté onions, add pureed tomatoes and garlic. Gradually stir in chili powder. Add cumin and oregano. Simmer for 30 minutes, stirring frequently. Makes 3 cups.

Use on tacos and enchiladas. If you leave out the cumin you can use it as a base for chicken, fish, or meat dishes.

MARINADE FOR MEAT

¼ cup red wine
2 T. mild soy sauce
¼ cup lime juice
½ cup chopped green pepper
½ cup chopped red pepper
½ cup chopped onion
¼ t. black pepper
1 T. Worcestershire sauce
½ t. garlic powder
½ t. onion powder
1 T. dry mustard

FROZEN BANANA SANDWICH

Serves 2

ripe banana
specially prepared peanut butter

Slice banana lengthwise, then in half. Spread 1 T. specially prepared peanut butter between two halves, close, wrap and freeze.

PAT'S NO-CRUST APPLE PIE

pippin apples, cored and sliced, 1 per person
1 t. vanilla
lemon juice
cinnamon, to taste
Sweet 'n Low brown-sugar

Cook sliced apples in a pan with vanilla, Sweet 'n Low, lemon juice (just a little) and cinnamon until done. Leave them a little bit crunchy.

RHUBARB DESSERT

Serves 6

2 packages frozen rhubarb, unsweetened
2 cans strawberry Shasta diet drink
1 can creme Shasta diet drink
1 package cranberries (optional)

Mix the rhubarb and Shasta drinks together in a pan and boil for 3 minutes. In a separate pan, add to cranberries just enough water to cover them and boil until they pop. Add them to the rhubarb mixture and cook for 3 minutes. Chill and serve.

SPICE LIST

These spices are good with these foods.

SHELLFISH	SEASONED SAUCES	FRUIT	SALAD DRESSING
anise	allspice	anise	anise
basil	basil	caraway seed	bay leaf

Hit the Spot Recipes

bay leaf	bon appétit	cinnamon	cardamom
curry powder	cardamom	cloves	chili powder
dill	cayenne pepper	coriander	ginger
garlic	chili powder	fennel	garlic
marjoram	cloves	ginger	marjoram
onion	coriander	mace	mustard
	curry powder	poppy seed	pepper
	dill	pumpkin	season all
	fennel	pie spice	tarragon
	garlic	rosemary	turmeric
	ginger	vanilla	
	mustard		
	nutmeg		
	oregano		
	parsley		
	savory		

BEEF	VEAL	LAMB	FISH
allspice	allspice	curry powder	anise
basil	cumin	garlic	bay leaf
bon appétit	curry powder	ginger	celery seed
cloves	garlic	mace	coriander
coriander	ginger	marjoram	curry powder
cumin	marjoram	mint	dill
curry powder	poultry seasoning	oregano	fennel seed
garlic	season all	rosemary	garlic
ginger	tarragon	season all	herb seasoning
herb seasoning			mace
mace			marjoram
marjoram			onion
mustard			paprika
onion			parsley
paprika			pepper
parsley			rosemary
sage			saffron
savory			sage
season all			season all
			tarragon
			turmeric

VEGETABLES	PASTA	EGGS	POULTRY
basil	basil	basil	bon appétit
bon appétit	caraway seed	bon appétit	chili powder
caraway seeds	celery seed	celery seed	cumin
celery seeds	chili powder	cumin	curry powder
chili powder	cinnamon	curry powder	garlic
cinnamon	cumin	dill	ginger
cloves	dill	mustard	herb seasoning
cumin	ginger	onion	mace
curry powder	oregano	oregano	marjoram
dill		paprika	mustard
ginger		pepper, cayenne	onion
garlic			paprika
herb seasoning		poppy seed	parsley
mace		savory	poultry seasoning
marjoram		season all	rosemary
mint		turmeric	saffron
mustard			sage
nutmeg			season all
poppy seed			tarragon
season all			turmeric
thyme			

MARINADES	CHEESE	DIPS	POTATOES
basil	bon appétit	bon appétit	caraway seed
caraway seed	caraway seed	celery seed	dill
cumin	chili powder	chili powder	garlic
curry powder	cumin	cumin	
garlic	dill	curry powder	
pepper	fennel	dill	
rosemary	garlic	garlic	
sage		mustard	
tarragon			

SOUPS	BREADS
cinnamon	garlic
coriander	caraway seed
garlic	dill
bay leaf	
pepper	
tarragon	
onion	
saffron	

THE SPOT REDUCING DIET AS A WAY OF LIFE

15

DINING OUT

You may dine out any place, even in a pizza parlor, if it has a salad bar, though some restaurants should not be visited more than once a month. See individual listings, p. 175, for recommendations.

While you're hitting the spot you must be acutely aware of everything you put into your mouth—beverages as well as food. Restaurant food is often loaded with hidden ingredients—butter, oil, flour, corn starch, salt, MSG, sugar—things that often do more to enhance your spots than to enhance the flavor or the food.

The trick to dining out while you are losing weight is knowing what to order and how to order it. Halibut, a lean fish, can be painted with melted butter before it hits the grill and basted with even more oil while it's cooking. By the time it reaches you, a lean fish has become a fatty and therefore a fattening fish. Tell the waiter you want your fish *broiled without oil or fat*. Otherwise you may be getting far more than your daily allotment of fat without even knowing it.

Take your dining-out cues from the restaurant listings. Follow the yeses and avoid the nos. There are literally dozens of choices. There's no reason for you to be bored or to feel deprived while you're hitting your spots. When you're finished, *voilà!* You will be able to eat anything you can control. Even dessert.

Food Sense

Pureed vegetables are usually a tender, colorful medium for cream, butter, salt, even sugar. Restaurant ratatouilli, unlike mine, is loaded with oil. Thick sauces are thickened with flour and cornstarch, two ingredients that will keep your waistline from shrinking.

Many of the gourmets I know think the more they get into exotic sauces and exotic foods the more gourmet they are. To me, the true gourmet is one who enjoys the *essence* of fine food. It takes a very fine veal chop to be served naked. It takes only a mediocre veal shop to be served under a blanket of thick, rich sauce.

Give your taste buds a treat. Allow them to savor the delicious essences of foods and before long you'll be able to isolate and identify ingredients simply by taste. If a dish is loaded with fat or salt or sugar, you'll taste it immediately. Your food sense will become more and more keen until you will automatically be able to make good food choices.

Some of my clients think that getting over sugar addiction and fat addiction is analogous to giving up smoking. The craving for a cigarette is overwhelming every once in a while but one's satisfaction with being able to breathe and to smell well far outweighs a moment's craving. Once you've become accustomed to tasting the essence of food it won't take more than a few bites to satisfy a craving. Clients on Maintenance find that bingeing on foods loaded with fat, salt, or sugar will make them sick. Just as with a reformed smoker, the best reward is feeling 100 percent healthier.

Bobby Colomby, formerly the drummer with Blood, Sweat and Tears, is now a record executive and record producer. He came to me to lose weight all over. He loved junk food. It took the six-footer about three months to lose 50 pounds and to develop good food sense. No more eating a mocha cake for breakfast and chocolate chip cookies as they came out of the oven so that he could make the next batch.

Bobby has kept his weight stable for three years and I suspect that armed with the knowledge, physique, and energy he's gained as a result of balancing his nutrients he will never be fat again. "I don't need goo anymore," he says. "I would rather have breast of chicken with a few spices than with heavy sauce all over it. Spices are, after all, the things that go into sauces to make them taste good."

In restaurants he asks that his food be prepared without salt. "I ask what's in the sauce," he says emphatically. "And I don't stand for evasive answers. It behooves a restaurant to be accommodating about food preparation because they know if they are you'll come back, and that's what they're there for."

Casey Kasem and his lovely wife, Jean, both hit their spots while dining out almost every night. Casey is a vegetarian so it is imperative that he have his vegetables. Jean discovered how easy it was to get food prepared the way she and Casey wanted it. "I think restaurants almost enjoy your asking for something steamed," she says. "Casey gets fantastic vegetables served to him that aren't even on the menu. I don't think anybody minds your asking that the sauce be left off or put on the side."

Don't Be Afraid to Ask!

Ask and you shall receive your food without hidden ingredients. The best, most painless and effective method of getting exactly what you want—what you should be having—is to call the restaurant ahead of time.

Tell the person in charge or the maître d' that you are not allowed to have oil or sugar in your food and what would he suggest you order? Be polite, but if the person happens to give you a hard time, simply say, "It's doctor's order. I suffer from hypertension." Or, "I'm diabetic and I can't have sugar and have to watch my fat." In my experience that little white lie will engender cooperation without further explanation. Saying you are on a diet to lose weight may only irritate the management instead of getting you the information and the food you want.

On occasion I've called restaurants that have been honest enough to say that everything is prepared in advance and it all has oil in it, so don't bother coming. And if that's the case, you're much better off going to a different restaurant until you're ready for Maintenance.

Ninety percent of the time, if you ask a restaurant to broil a chicken breast or fish without butter or oil, they will be happy to do it. If they don't have steamed vegetables on the menu, ask for them anyway. If they can't accommodate you, eat the vegetables you missed when you get home.

When Gloria Harvey, a beautiful middle-aged woman, first came to me, she was top-heavy but she also wanted to slim down all over. "I don't think I can follow this, Hermien. My husband and I are going to New York for a week. We'll be eating every meal in a restaurant."

"That doesn't make any difference," I told her. "You can go to any restaurant and get food prepared the way you want it. Take your specially prepared peanut butter and the Laughing Cow cheese wedges just to be safe."

Gloria came back from Manhattan two pounds lighter and a lot wiser. She learned how little effort it really does take to get what you want. "We went to Twenty-One," she said, "and I wanted to order my favorite dinner, soft-shelled crab, but I knew I shouldn't. When the waiter came to take our order I said, 'I'd like the soft-shelled crab but I can't have anything with butter or grease.' He asked me how I would like it prepared. I said, 'Broiled without oil.' He said, 'Fine.' I got my soft-shelled crab broiled without oil and it was absolutely delicious. My husband even enjoyed it that way.

"Then, when we came back to Los Angeles we had dinner at an excellent fish restaurant. I asked for soft-shelled crab broiled without butter. The waiter spoke to the chef, who said he couldn't make them that way because they'd fall apart. I said, 'I don't care if they fall apart. I can't have butter or grease because it makes me sick. I'll take my chances and have them broiled.' They didn't fall apart and now every time I go to the place the waiter says, 'Yes, you're the lady who wants broiled soft-shell crabs without butter.' "

Gloria lost 32 pounds without having to give up the food she loves or the pleasures of dining out. She's no longer top-heavy; she is maintaining her perfectly proportioned figure.

The Dinner Party

Dining out at other people's homes can be especially tricky. You don't want to offend them by refusing their homemade hospitality but you don't want to wear it on your stomach or your thighs for the next three weeks either.

Suzanne Somers trimmed her saddlebags and beautifully balanced her figure nearly ten years ago. She and her husband, Alan Hamel, dine out nearly every night. And Suzanne, a gourmet cook, knows how sensitive people are who've spent days, sometimes, preparing a special lunch or dinner. If you're going to a large dinner party Suzanne suggests, "If it's dinner for twelve, you can scrape the breading off and just eat the chicken and talk a lot. I request water as soon as we sit down. I just ask for more and more water so they don't see that I'm not drinking the wine. I know how annoying it is when you have someone over who won't eat what you've prepared for them, so I try not to let them know."

In a smaller group you can still take a few polite bites and leave the rest. Say you're not hungry or you don't like or are allergic to one of the key ingredients. For example if the main course was lasagna you might say, "I love lasagna, it's one of my favorite dishes, especially the way you make it, but lately I've been having a strange reaction to dairy products—there's cheese in lasagna—so I don't want to eat too much tonight."

Your objective is to take the pressure off yourself without hurting your hostess's feelings. If you say you've had a sensitive stomach that day no one will take it personally.

Naturally, if you're among close friends and can tell them you're on a special slimming, spot reducing diet that's ideal. It's the other situations, in which you may be embarrassed or uncomfortable or worry about hurting someone's feelings, that a little white lie will keep you on the right spot reducing track. If you don't follow the daily balance of protein, fat, and carbohydrate you will not achieve a well balanced shape. And if you've hit your spots and then return to your old eating habits your body will return to its former disproportionate shape.

Conventions, Banquets, and Big Celebrations

When a meal has been prearranged at a hotel or a restaurant, it is possible to call ahead to make special eating arrangements. For anyone with a physical problem such as diabetes or hypertension, calling in advance is common practice. Restaurants are used to special requests, so don't be afraid to call. Try them the day before the affair, if possible.

June and Marvin Disney are two former clients who have consistently maintained their slim, balanced shapes. They attribute their continued success to *planning ahead*. When they go to a charity or political dinner they never leave anything to chance. June says, "I always call the hotel the day before or the morning of the banquet and inquire about the menu. If it's something we can't eat—something breaded or swimming in oil—I order either broiled chicken or fish and I give them our table number. And there's no problem. In fact, everybody else at the table is aggravated because they'd rather be eating what we're eating."

There are certain restrictions during the program, but remember, when you're finished you'll be able to eat anything you can control. That means that on Maintenance you will have guidelines to keep yourself from overeating. And if you stay within those guidelines, you can eat any food you want, or drink any beverage in moderation. Moderation for a man 6'4" tall is different from moderation for a 5'2" woman. It is a level that each individual must discover for himself or herself.

Tips for Dining Out

Never go to a restaurant or a party when you're hungry.
  If you're going from home, have a bowl of Hit the Spot ratatouille or vegetable soup just before leaving. If you're going from the office, open a can of uncut string beans or asparagus. Always keep a few cans of food you can eat nearby. Also a can opener. That will make the spot-reducing process easier and more enjoyable.

Plan ahead. Know what you're going to order. Don't look at the menu!
  Again, if you know where you will be dining out, telephone the restaurant the day of your impending visit and ask if they have anything on their menu that is broiled, baked, boiled, or roasted without butter or oil. Tell them that for health reasons it's best if you find out ahead of time. And always be polite. If they give you a hard time, tell them you would really like to go there and you hope there's something you can eat. Ninety percent of the time they will be helpful.
  The reason I recommend not looking at the menu is that it's too easy to order what sounds good instead of what you should be having. It's too tempting to order a dish described poetically instead of a broiled chicken breast.

Make adjustments for hidden ingredients.
If you're going to be eating food you know contains oil or fat, flour, cornstarch, sugar, or honey, *leave off your bread and butter for that day.* If you go to a restaurant on the spur of the moment and think that you've had more than your daily allotment of fat, *leave off 1 oz. of fat for the next two days.* If you're going to a dinner party, cut down on breakfast and lunch that day. Have:
Breakfast: 1 egg and 1 piece of fruit
Lunch: ⅔ cup lowfat cottage cheese

Weights
If you eat exclusively in restaurants, be sure that you are meeting your daily spot-reducing Master Plan requirements. Buy a food scale and measuring cups. Use them at home so that you will know what 4 ounces of cooked meat looks like versus anything more or less. You can always buy a specified number of ounces of turkey breast or lean roast beef at a deli.

Vegetables
If you can't get enough vegetables to satisfy the daily requirement: It seems that the most difficult thing to do for someone who eats out a lot is to get three cups of vegetables a day. The easiest answer is to *eat what you missed when you get home.* Even if you are a busy executive you can still buy fresh, frozen, or canned vegetables. It's the vegetables that give you the glow that radiates good health.

Don't eat less than the daily requirements!
If you think you will lose weight faster by eating *less* than I've specified on the Master Plan, you will lose pounds without changing your shape or losing your spots. The key to spot reducing is eating the right balance of nutrients and allowing your body to reproportion itself slowly.

Drinking
You may have 1 4-oz. glass of dry white wine or 1 oz. of hard liquor instead of that day's bread allotment. Never both or your spots from the waist up won't shrink. *No juice of any kind* while you're hitting your spots. Drink Perrier or Poland water, plain water, coffee, tea, or diet soda.

Bread and rolls
   You may eat the *crust only*. Unless, of course, you're having your daily bread allotment. As for butter, none unless you want to count it as part of that day's allowance.

Dessert
   There is no reason why you have to feel deprived while you're losing weight. Be smart, save one serving of fruit or make strawberry cloud when you get home. I've included a bedtime snack on each day's menu so that when you dine out you will have something to look forward to when you get home. That will make watching everyone eat his dessert far less tedious. And in the long run, losing your spots will be more delicious than any dessert you've ever tasted. I guarantee it!

What to do at a pizza parlor
   If the pizza parlor has a salad bar or you know you can order a salad without garbanzo beans and salami chunks, fine. I've had good luck with clients who have planned ahead when going to a pizza parlor by bringing a Baggie with turkey cut in fingers or chicken breast in bite-sized pieces. Place your protein on top of the salad and you've gotten everything you need. Most pizza parlors don't have protein available that you can eat. Plan ahead!

Always fork-prong your salad dressing.
   Again, always order salad dressing *on the side*. Never dip your salad into the dressing or your spots from the waist down will never disappear.

Never order anything broasted or fried.
   "Broasted" can mean the food has been fried before roasting. Fried food is always loaded with fat.

When dining out, keep a lookout for the following—they're the biggest offenders:
   bread and butter
   hors d'oeuvres
   chips and dips
   alcoholic beverages
   nuts
   olives

fried, breaded, creamed foods
salad with dressing *not on the side*
pureed vegetables
cream and sugar
salt
MSG
sherbet
Parmesan cheese toast and garlic bread
low-calorie desserts—generally high in both flour and fat
salami
garbanzo beans
frozen yogurt—high in sugar

AVOID:
    looking at a beautiful menu with provocative descriptions
    going hungry
    being bullied by a waiter or waitress
    food that accompanies what you've ordered
    cheating!

Restaurant Guide to Dining Out

Yes, you can still enjoy your favorite ethnic restaurants. Here's a rundown on the acceptable delicacies and potential dangers of each specialty.

AMERICAN

ENJOY: fish (from lean list)
              chicken (white meat, no skin)
              turkey (white meat, no skin)
              meat (from lean list)
              small baked potato, no sour cream
              vegetable salad
              steamed vegetables

AVOID: fried, breaded, or broasted anything

CHINESE

ENJOY:
egg drop soup
hot and sour soup
chicken chop suey
chicken and shrimp and Chinese vegetables, or chicken or shrimp and snow peas or broccoli
chicken Zechuan
beef dish—counts as one of your two allowed for the week
½ cup steamed rice
(If you don't have rice you can have one slice of bread during the day.)

AVOID:
nuts, moo shu anything, glass noodles or other noodles
fried rice or fried anything
egg rolls
ribs
rumaki
seeds
pork

CONTINENTAL

ENJOY:
broiled or baked fish from lean-fish list
chicken breast
turkey breast
small filet mignon
lamb or seafood en brochette
steamed vegetables
vegetable salad
veal or chicken paillard

AVOID:
anything accompanied by a sauce containing oil, butter, flour, animal drippings, or cream

DELICATESSEN

ENJOY:
scrambled eggs
scrambled eggs with onions
omelet (always 2-egg, never 3)
mushroom omelet

chicken liver omelet
salads—hard-boiled eggs and cottage cheese
stuffed tomato with tuna or turkey salad
broiled hamburger
tuna salad sandwich (white meat tuna)
roast turkey sandwich (white meat)
turkey salad sandwich
roast beef (if you want to use it as one of
 your two beef meals for the week)
beet borscht—without sour cream
whole wheat or rye bagel

If you order a sandwich, ask for rye or whole wheat bread with mustard unless you want to use your fat allotment for the day.

AVOID: herring
whitefish
salmon (lox)
kippers
tongue
pastrami
corned beef
cod
sturgeon
matzo balls
gefilte fish
pumpernickel bagels
bagel chips
potato salad
marinated anything

ENGLISH

ENJOY: roast beef, lean
roast turkey breast
steamed vegetables
fresh fruit salad

AVOID: roast potatoes
Welsh rarebit
vegetables cooked alongside meat
steak and kidney pie
shepherd's pie
fish and chips

trifle
bread and butter pudding

FRENCH

ENJOY:
consommé
bouillabaisse if not oil-based
fish or chicken broiled dry with lemon, herbs, and/or wine or all three
tenderloin broiled with wine (no fat)
brochette of seafood, fish, white chicken, or turkey
baked potato
salad—fork-prong dressing
steamed vegetables
fresh fruit

AVOID:
puree
baked *stuffed* potato
bread or butter the day you go
cream sauces
fatty cheese
flour-based sauces

GERMAN

ENJOY:
steamed vegetables, broiled or grilled fish or poultry
salad with dressing on the side

AVOID: Most German food; it's high in fat, so beware.

While on the Spot Reducing Diet do not have German cuisine more than once a month.

HEALTH FOOD

ENJOY:
2-egg omelet with vegetables
salad
fresh fruit with cottage cheese or plain lowfat yogurt
Be sure to have at least 2 oz. of protein for lunch, so if you order a salad that's only vegetables, have a side order of cottage cheese.

The Spot Reducing Diet as a Way of Life

AVOID: avocado
nuts
dried fruits
more than 1 oz. of cheese
frozen yogurt
carrot cake

INDIAN

ENJOY: fish kebab
vegetable kebab
chicken tandoori
lamb tandoori
tikka—chunks without bones
lamb curry
½ cup rice

AVOID: anything made with oil

Be sure to leave bread and butter off the day you go. While on the Spot Reducing Diet do not have Indian cuisine more than once a month.

ITALIAN

ENJOY: veal marsala or veal scallopini—but must
not be breaded or fried
broiled veal chop or broiled seafood
½ cup plain spaghetti or 1 bread crust
from 1 slice bread
Italian antipasto—peppers, tomatoes,
pickles, and greens
chicken cacciatore
fresh fruit

AVOID: bread or butter that day
marinara, piccata, Parmesan
antipasto with oil
garbanzo beans
olives
salami
anchovies

breaded veal or chicken dishes
anything Alfredo
pesto

JAPANESE

ENJOY:
miso soup
sashimi
fish or chicken steamed in soy or water
Japanese vegetables
cucumber—no dressing
fresh fruit

AVOID:
sushi
teryaki—it has brown sugar
sukyaki—it has white sugar
tempura
bread or butter that day

MEXICAN

ENJOY:
one small corn tortilla instead of bread
    (small corn tortilla has 55 cals.; flour 90)
hot sauce
chicken tostada—tortilla on bottom should
    not be eaten
chicken, lettuce, chopped tomatoes, their
    tostada sauce and a little cheese
2-egg Spanish omelet
Spanish chicken if not fried or breaded
Mexican salad—your dressing or fork-
    prong dressing
fresh fruit

AVOID:
flour tortilla
chips or dip
avocado
sour cream
beans
margaritas

SEAFOOD

ENJOY:
broiled or baked fish
bouillabaisse—if not oil-based
cioppino—if not oil-based
red chowder—if no oil in it
If you have something broiled, ask that it be cooked with lemon juice, *not* fat or oil.
mixed green salad
baked potato or ½ cup rice
steamed vegetables
fresh fruit

AVOID:
anything fried or that has oil
fatty fish

THAI

It has been my experience that it is difficult to find any dishes on a Thai menu that don't contain either oil, sugar, or MSG; therefore, while you're on the program it is best to avoid Thai cuisine. Save it for Maintenance.

16

TRAVEL

"Taste the delicacies of the Orient."
"Play today—pay tomorrow!"
"Enjoy French cuisine as only the French can prepare it."
"Eat, drink, and be merry" is the plea the travel industry likes to put forth. And why not? It's the lure of breathtaking sunsets and exotic foods that seduces most of us into traveling. And more likely than not, your family album features plenty of your favorite mouth-watering moments. Eating is more memorable than sights you've seen. Food is always on your mind. Please don't leave home without your *food sense*.

You know what caused your spots; you know how to lose them—or if you've lost them, how to keep them from ever returning. You can eat anything you can control. If you know yourself well enough to know that one taste will lead to infinity, don't take that first bite.

This chapter will give you enough travel tips to guide you through almost any difficult situation. The key is to *plan ahead*. You'll discover that temptation lurks around every cloud, whistle-stop, and safe harbor.

Your Body Doesn't Know You're on Vacation

Your body doesn't care if you're at home, on the beach in Hawaii, or on a perch nestled in the Swiss Alps. As many of my clients have discovered, if you give yourself permission to eat it, you'll wear it. I tell people this over and over, and the ones who don't believe me come home with souvenir *spots*.

Joy Philbin came to me to trim her thighs. She hit that spot for less than six weeks and finally had a perfectly proportioned figure. She and Regis went off to Mexico for a vacation. "When Regis and I arrived in Mexico I had a perfect figure. We started with margaritas and the enchiladas and all the wonderful Mexican cooking and by the third or fourth day I looked entirely different in my bathing suit. Regis spotted it right away. He said, 'You've lost your perfect figure—it's gone!'

"I was so sad. I found out if I ate a lot of meat and fried food the fat would go right to my thighs. I saw it happen in a week's time. When I got home I went back on the program. The Spot Reducing Diet's not a diet, it's a way of life. It's made me understand my body—where certain foods and drinks—go. I really pay attention now. It doesn't matter if I'm at home or on vacation; I prefer thin legs to a few chips and a bowl of guacamole."

Planes

If you're going by plane and a meal is to be served, tell your travel agent or the airline's ticket agent that you are on a special diet and you must order your meal before boarding. This is common practice, so don't be shy.

Order a seafood salad, a low-calorie plate, or fresh fruit with cottage cheese. If more than one meal is to be served, place your order for that as well. If you haven't preordered you may find yourself with very fattening entrée choices.

One problem is that people often make substitutions that are convenient but not comparable. For example, eating a serving of lasagna and omitting your bread for that day may or may not be a fair exchange. You may be getting twice the amount of bread you are supposed to have without even realizing it. Then you wonder why your belt is getting tight. The same formula is true for the fat or oil content in many dishes. You may think you've brushed the fat off but instead you may find yourself sitting on it.

TYPICAL PLANE FARE

ENJOY: diet drinks
mineral water (Perrier or Poland water)
coffee or tea
plain water—One has a tendency to become dehydrated while flying. To help minimize jet lag, drink one small glass of water every half hour.

AVOID: fruit juice
wine and alcohol
nuts and cheese
pretzels and crackers

Casey Kasem spends most of his time on the air but when he and Jean are in the air they plan their own meals. "When we fly," Jean explains, "we take a picnic of toasted bread sliced in little squares. I use the very thin sliced bread. I cut the squares the same size as the cheese. We use Laughing Cow Green Label. We carry our own diet drinks because I've discovered that even when you ask for a diet drink they may give you one with sugar. Also, taking a picnic is very romantic. When we're flying we don't get interrupted so we get a chance to spend time together."

Another couple who've made the Spot Reducing Diet a way of life is Victoria and Ed McMahon. Victoria explained, "What I try to do is take our own food aboard the aircraft. Because when you're sitting there it's a natural thing to want to eat. And it's not necessarily something you want—it's just that it's there and it looks good and so you have it. Knowing that, I plan ahead. I will broil a turkey breast and take sliced turkey. I will take a chicken breast or cold lobster, one of Ed's favorites."

On the plane the McMahons enjoy their own picnic. When they reach their destination they are able to order what they want from room service. "Most hotels have a nice little picnic basket," Victoria mentioned. "They have a broiled chicken or at least they're happy to prepare it. Normally they will make something for us. I sometimes travel with low-calorie Laughing Cow cheese."

The same plane tips apply to train food.

Beware the Continental Breakfast

The world over, hotels and even some motels offer a complimentary Continental breakfast. That usually means a glass of orange juice, which contains sugar from three oranges and enhances your spots from the waist up, a sweet roll or a croissant, which is loaded with butter and some sugar.

The fat and sugar content of a typical Continental breakfast is an open invitation to giving yourself *permission*. Breakfast is only the first meal of the day and somehow one little bite makes you feel as if you've blown it for the rest of the day. It's easy to *decide to start tomorrow*—but tomorrow never comes. Remember: it's the first bite that makes you feel the fattest. One crunch and you'll feel you've blown it. Even if it's free—if it's spot-producing or fattening, forget it. Instead, be ready with a Laughing Cow cheese wedge and a piece of fruit or a small can of fruit in its own juice. Read the label! Substitute foods you know you can have.

Early in the morning or late in the afternoon when you've had a long, exhausting day and you need a lift, or even before bed—be prepared. Have the right foods with you. You'll feel better during your trip and you'll look better when you get home.

Your Limitations

Before you leave on your trip, decide on your limitations. If it makes you unhappy to do that, you must accept the fact that if you eat it, you'll wear it.

Actress Julie Carmen came to me several years ago to reproportion her body and learn good nutrition. She was a young dancer with a passion for cheese. She had big thighs from the fat food she was eating. Her face was a little too round from eating too much bread and pasta. We went to work and Julie hit all her spots. She lost 20 pounds and has kept them off because she knows her limitations.

She spent five months in hotels in 1982. "I spent three months filming in West Berlin and two months in Florida and Puerto Rico. I know how difficult it is to keep your weight down, feel satisfied and get all your nutrients when you're on the road. To make sure that I have what I need I take:

3 Tupperware containers (2 medium-sized and 1 small one)
a potato peeler
a can opener
a small strainer
ziploc storage bags
paper towels

"I used to carry an old bathroom scale and my blender. In Germany I discovered nonfat Speisequark, a yogurty cheese that has very little fat. I bought frozen vegetables and thawed them in my Tupperware. The hardest thing to do on the road is get your vegetables. In Europe they don't have many places where you can buy prepared food to go. Italian restaurants in Germany will make things for you without oil. I'd go to the same restaurant every day. That made it easier to get what I needed."

Julie solved the problem of eating bread, rolls, or crackers on an airplane by taking raw vegetables with her. "Whenever I'm bored—an eighteen-hour flight can get pretty boring—I eat raw vegetables. While everyone else is eating nuts and crackers and cheese, I'm chewing on carrot sticks. I carry food with me so that I have what I want on the flight as well as when I arrive. Planning ahead is the best insurance. I take pop-top cans of tuna packed in water (pour the water out, using your small strainer), Laughing Cow Green Label cheese, specially prepared peanut butter, which I fix at home, measure into one-tablespoon servings and pack in individual Ziploc storage bags, instant miso soup and a small amount of nonfat powdered milk. When I arrive I buy: spring water, decaffeinated coffee, cinnamon, and vanilla. Knowing just how compulsive I can be about food, I keep my bags of peanut butter locked inside a duffel bag. To get it out I have to go to all the trouble of unlocking the padlock. I have to *think* before I eat it."

Having adopted the Spot Reducing Diet as a way of life, Suzanne Somers and Alan Hamel *plan ahead.*

"We bring a jar of deoiled peanut butter and we buy apples. That's a normal breakfast. We order tea and some toast. If we don't have peanut butter, we might have an egg. We always pay attention to nutritional balance."

Both Suzanne and Alan learned to really *taste* their food. In restaurants anywhere in the world, if you discover that the food has a lot of grease or flour, Suzanne suggests, "You eat around it. If you're on the road six months of the year as I am, and if you eat only the food available in restaurants, it will catch up with you. So, if we're on the road for a long period of time we bring our own kitchen.

"We keep a case with a wok and a rice steamer, an electric frying pan just so that at some point during the day I can have something to eat that's going to give me a lot of energy."

When traveling abroad the Hamels have learned to appreciate the cuisine without wearing it home. They seek out seafood restaurants. "Even in Europe," Suzanne said, "you can get seafood without sauce. You have to ask! Shellfish, steamed clams, things like that. In Europe you learn to work around the fattening cuisine and at the same time not deny yourself one of the greatest pleasures—food. If I eat something and it has a lot of hidden fat in it it'll make me sick. My body just can't handle it now, thank goodness!"

Always remember: *When you know your limitations* and you're on Maintenance, *you'll be able to eat anything you can control.*

The Polite "No, Thank You!"

When traveling, the safest policy is to let your host know beforehand that you're on a special diet. That will make life more comfortable for everybody.

You must learn to be polite but *firm*. Tell the person—*confide in him*—that you've been to the doctor and she's told you to watch your sugar and fat for a few weeks. Once you've stated that as fact, you won't be able to give yourself permission to eat anything *more than your daily allotment* of those items. Nor will your host be compelled to insist that you do. If you don't set the scene from the beginning, you won't have a chance.

There is, however, always the person who refuses to take "no" for an answer. If Aunt Lizzie knows that her chocolate coconut cake has been your favorite since childhood she may feel that your polite "No, thank you" is a rejection of her and not simply the ingredients in her luscious cake. She places her masterpiece in front of you—you're on vacation—there's a fork pulsating next to your left hand—what are you going to do?

1. Tell Aunt Lizzie how wonderful it was of her to have gone to all the trouble of making your favorite dessert. Rave about the cake and say that you hope everyone else enjoys it. If Aunt Lizzie persists, say, "It's too bad I can't have it this year. I'll be back next year!" If you can do this, there is nothing in your life that you won't be able to control. Reward yourself later with anything other than food or drink. If it's your favorite dessert, you probably wouldn't be able to stop after that first crunch. If you succumb to Aunt Lizzie's emotional cue, you're in real trouble. Coconut cake is so full of empty calories you run the risk of hitting every spot in the wrong direction.
2. Think of something that will keep Aunt Lizzie from being terribly hurt—buy her a gift!—but don't hurt yourself by eating something because it's there.
3. Begin to think of eating sensibly as being good to yourself. If you do binge one day, don't undereat the next. Just delete the bread and alcohol. It doesn't matter which city you're in. This rule always applies.

Travel Tips

Take with you:
    specially prepared peanut butter (with paper towels)
    Laughing Cow Green Label cheese wedges
    tuna packed in water in pop-top cans (or take a can opener)

None of these things requires refrigeration. And if you're going abroad or even to another city in the United States where you're not certain whether or not you can get these items, be safe—carry a supply with you. You can always buy fresh fruit and vegetables from a local market or stand. In a foreign country it might be wise to get fruit with an outer skin that you peel off.

17

PREGNANCY

Being pregnant can be the most exciting time of your life—*if you feel well*. It is not a time to diet to lose weight. It is a time when it's especially important to eat the right balance and variety of nutrients, and all in moderation. The health of an expectant mother is directly related to the health of her baby.

It's easy to lose sight of your whole body when you're pregnant. The natural tendency is to focus on your ever-expanding midriff and to rationalize any other bulges. Maternity clothes help you block out and hide new lumps and bumps.

When my coauthor, Linda Lane, first came to me she wanted to get rid of her writer's rump. She was bottom-heavy and assumed it was a result of sitting at the typewriter for too long. Her backside was broad and she had saddlebags, but neither spot was related to sitting or typing. Linda was a fat addict. She loved butter-rich sauces, avocados, cheese, all parts of chicken and turkey, especially the crisp skin and dark meat. Dark meat contains more fat than white meat; skin, crispy or not, is mostly fat.

Linda spent two months hitting those spots; learning what caused them and how to avoid getting them back in the future. For the first time since her late teens she had a perfectly proportioned figure. She looked slim in tight French jeans.

Two years later, Linda was married and expecting her first baby.

"When I was five months pregnant, Hermien took one look at

me and said, 'Linda, you've gone back to your old eating habits. You probably can't see it but you're getting a big behind.' She poked at my rapidly refilling saddlebags and told me that if I didn't stop being a fat addict I was going to be even more bottom-heavy than before. It amazed me that she could look at me in a full, free-flowing garment and see that I'd reverted to eating dressing on my salad, sour cream on my baked potato, avocado in my salad, and drinking whole milk. My doctor had given me a special prenatal vitamin but he'd also told me I needed plenty of calcium, and milk was an excellent source. I told Hermien she was right but I felt I needed everything I was eating. I wasn't eating ice cream or desserts. I didn't think I'd reverted back too far."

" 'Vitamin A- and D-fortified nonfat milk has ninety calories in eight ounces, 2 percent lowfat contains 140 calories in eight ounces, and whole milk contains 150 calories in eight ounces. The only difference,' she insisted, 'between nonfat and the whole milk is a lot of extra *fat* calories. You don't need that extra fat and neither does your baby! Follow the Spot Reducing Diet, balance your nutrients and add one quart of vitamin A- and D-fortified nonfat milk a day. Then you'll be fine and you won't end up with a billboard behind and saddlebags.'

"Fortunately for me I knew Hermien was right. I switched from whole milk to the nonfat. I hated the chalky taste at first but I knew I'd rather make my taste buds suffer than spend a year trying to get rid of the lumps and bumps on my thighs, saddlebags, and behind. I gained about thirty pounds in nine months. My daughter is now four months old and I'm back into my old jeans. My husband is thrilled with our child and the way I look."

Eating properly will play a major role in helping you feel your best—having plenty of energy, feeling a sense of calm and well-being; even avoiding such complaints as constipation and indigestion. Both you and your baby *are what you eat*, so don't use pregnancy as an open-handed, open-mouthed ticket to food heaven. Remember: quality wins over quantity every time.

"Oh, Go On! You're Eating For Two!"

"You're eating for two" has to be the most overused appeal since "Start tomorrow!" It's true, you are eating for two—or more in some

17

PREGNANCY

Being pregnant can be the most exciting time of your life—*if you feel well*. It is not a time to diet to lose weight. It is a time when it's especially important to eat the right balance and variety of nutrients, and all in moderation. The health of an expectant mother is directly related to the health of her baby.

It's easy to lose sight of your whole body when you're pregnant. The natural tendency is to focus on your ever-expanding midriff and to rationalize any other bulges. Maternity clothes help you block out and hide new lumps and bumps.

When my coauthor, Linda Lane, first came to me she wanted to get rid of her writer's rump. She was bottom-heavy and assumed it was a result of sitting at the typewriter for too long. Her backside was broad and she had saddlebags, but neither spot was related to sitting or typing. Linda was a fat addict. She loved butter-rich sauces, avocados, cheese, all parts of chicken and turkey, especially the crisp skin and dark meat. Dark meat contains more fat than white meat; skin, crispy or not, is mostly fat.

Linda spent two months hitting those spots; learning what caused them and how to avoid getting them back in the future. For the first time since her late teens she had a perfectly proportioned figure. She looked slim in tight French jeans.

Two years later, Linda was married and expecting her first baby.

"When I was five months pregnant, Hermien took one look at

me and said, 'Linda, you've gone back to your old eating habits. You probably can't see it but you're getting a big behind.' She poked at my rapidly refilling saddlebags and told me that if I didn't stop being a fat addict I was going to be even more bottom-heavy than before. It amazed me that she could look at me in a full, free-flowing garment and see that I'd reverted to eating dressing on my salad, sour cream on my baked potato, avocado in my salad, and drinking whole milk. My doctor had given me a special prenatal vitamin but he'd also told me I needed plenty of calcium, and milk was an excellent source. I told Hermien she was right but I felt I needed everything I was eating. I wasn't eating ice cream or desserts. I didn't think I'd reverted back too far."

" 'Vitamin A- and D-fortified nonfat milk has ninety calories in eight ounces, 2 percent lowfat contains 140 calories in eight ounces, and whole milk contains 150 calories in eight ounces. The only difference,' she insisted, 'between nonfat and the whole milk is a lot of extra *fat* calories. You don't need that extra fat and neither does your baby! Follow the Spot Reducing Diet, balance your nutrients and add one quart of vitamin A- and D-fortified nonfat milk a day. Then you'll be fine and you won't end up with a billboard behind and saddlebags.'

"Fortunately for me I knew Hermien was right. I switched from whole milk to the nonfat. I hated the chalky taste at first but I knew I'd rather make my taste buds suffer than spend a year trying to get rid of the lumps and bumps on my thighs, saddlebags, and behind. I gained about thirty pounds in nine months. My daughter is now four months old and I'm back into my old jeans. My husband is thrilled with our child and the way I look."

Eating properly will play a major role in helping you feel your best—having plenty of energy, feeling a sense of calm and well-being; even avoiding such complaints as constipation and indigestion. Both you and your baby *are what you eat,* so don't use pregnancy as an open-handed, open-mouthed ticket to food heaven. Remember: quality wins over quantity every time.

"Oh, Go On! You're Eating For Two!"

"You're eating for two" has to be the most overused appeal since "Start tomorrow!" It's true, you are eating for two—or more in some cases—and your nutritional needs are greater, but you don't need additional calories. At least, not until the last three months, and then you'll need only an additional 10 to 20 percent—about 300 calories per day more than before you were pregnant.

If you give yourself permission to eat whatever you please without regard to its nutritional value, your body will reflect it. Don't think that because you're pregnant you can avoid filling up fat cells. If you eat foods loaded with fat, such as ice cream and whole milk, your posterior and thighs will bulge. I had one client who ate loads of fruit when she was pregnant and she got huge arms. Too much carbohydrate will make you fat from the waist up.

Play Chess with Food

Don't rely on vitamin and mineral supplements to give you everything you need. Your doctor may prescribe a prenatal vitamin. It's good insurance, but it can't possibly provide you with all the nutrients you and your baby need. Remember the eight amino acids that must be replenished on a daily basis. You'll be getting those when you eat *small* amounts of protein throughout the day, not from a vitamin pill.

Use your food scale. Make sure that you're having nine ounces of protein a day (if you're taller you might want to have ten ounces) *plus* one quart of vitamin A- and D-fortified nonfat milk. Space your meals out.

It should also be noted that playing doctor—thinking that if one vitamin is good, five are great—can be dangerous. Excess doses of vitamins can harm your baby. Play chess with your diet and get the full range of vitamins and minerals.

How you gain weight is as important as how much weight you gain. How much you gain will depend on your size, eating habits, general health, and your doctor's recommendation. Plan to gain between 20 and 30 pounds during the nine months. If your weight gain is more than expected, consult your doctor but never diet to lose weight. Your baby will triple in weight during the last three months, making your nutritional needs just that much greater. You are also building your milk supply during the third trimester.

I had one client, Mary, who was petite, 5'2" tall and boyishly built. That is, until she got pregnant and ate herself into blimpdom.

Both she and her husband were in their early twenties. They were young and too innocent to realize that Mary's largeness was not healthy for either mother or baby.

In her seventh month Mary looked as if she could deliver at any moment. I told her that even though she had gained far too much weight—she was big and fat all over from eating much too much protein—now was not the time to lose weight. I asked her how she had managed to go for so long without becoming alarmed by the changes to her whole body. She looked *swollen*.

"I don't know . . . I guess I thought you had to gain weight all over when you're pregnant. My mom gained 55 pounds with my younger sister. They're both okay."

"Do they have a weight problem—your mother and sister?"

"Yeah—they're always on a diet, but Mom used to be really skinny like I used to be. I've always eaten whatever I wanted—I've never had a weight problem till now. God, I'm uncomfortable!"

It seemed that Mary's husband indulged her food cravings day and night because he thought that food was the pregnant mother's reward. He'd been brought up on the old pickles and ice cream fantasy: if she craves it, give it to her because she *needs* it. But *nobody* needs hand-to-mouth disease!

A pregnant woman's nutrient needs are greater for certain vitamins and minerals: half again as much calcium, one-third more vitamin C, two-thirds more protein, one-quarter more riboflavin and vitamin A, one-third more vitamin B_{12}, twice as much folic acid, and more thiamine, niacin, and vitamins B_6, D, and E, as well as iron and other minerals. You need all those nutrients *but you need only 15 percent more calories* than before you were pregnant. Be sure to take a prenatal vitamin.

Calcium is especially important for building baby's strongbones and primary teeth. It also has a calming effect. The best way to get your daily calcium is by drinking one quart of vitamin A- and D-fortified nonfat milk: you need six to eight glasses of fluid a day, and milk is an excellent source of calcium and fluid.

By drinking nonfat milk you'll save over 200 calories a day. Think of it as an exchange. Exchange whole milk for nonfat and have two slices of wheat toast or a small banana and one tablespoon of specially prepared peanut butter or a variety of other foods. See the Exchange Lists for more alternatives. Be creative with meals. You

KATHARINE ROSS DEMONSTRATES SPOT REDUCING EXERCISES— AND HOW TO MEASURE THE RESULTS

Use this section along with Chapter 20, "Ron Fletcher's Exercise Guide"

Whole Body Toner

The whole body toner involves exactly what its name implies: feet, legs, posterior, stomach, spine and on up to the neck and the top of the head. Think of a string extending from the back of your head pulling you upward. (all photographs of Katharine Ross by Nancy Lee Andrews)

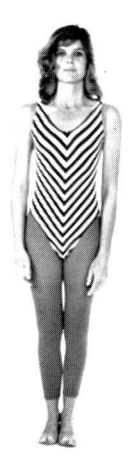
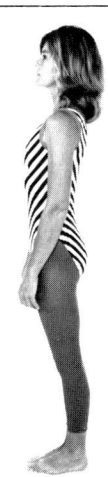

Stand straight: ankles touching, knees together. Lift your toes.

Flatten your toes and with ankles and knees together, *lengthen your body upward.* Concentrate first on the low abdominal muscles, then the ribs, then lift your sternum upward so that your neck will lengthen. When finished, your body should be aligned as Katharine's is in the photograph.

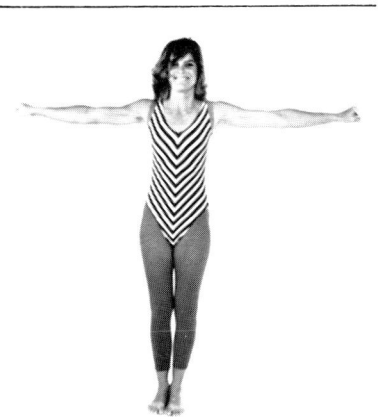
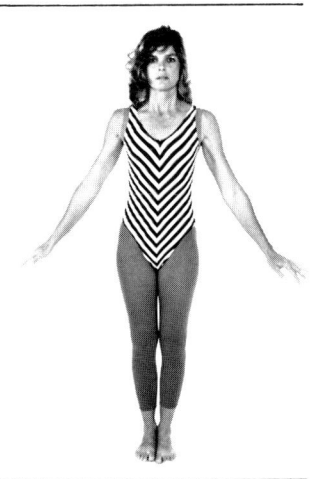

Extend your arms up and out to your sides, parallel to the floor. Make a fist and take a deep breath. Contract your buttocks. Raise your eyebrows.

Repeat this exercise for 10 minutes twice a day.

Release. Relax and begin again.

Body Lift

This slow, careful exercise will use up more energy than you think, and involves total mind/body involvement.

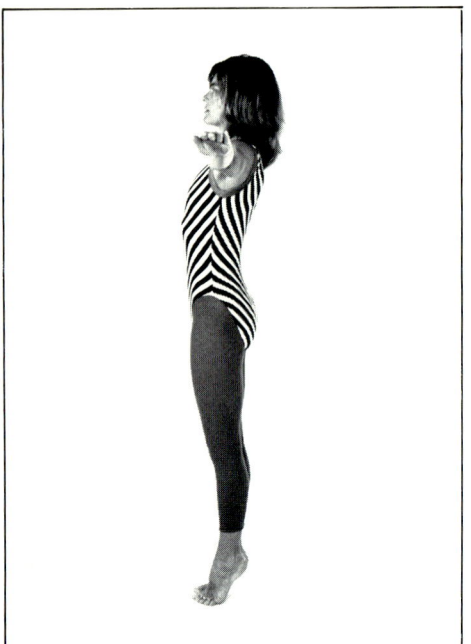

Stand tall with body aligned as in the *Whole Body Toner*. Contract buttocks muscles. Lift up onto your toes. Extend arms to the side. Lift up and come down. Take a deep breath on the way up—letting it out as you come down.

Be sure that you are balancing over the center toes. Do not roll to the outside of your feet. Your body should look like Katharine's.

Begin by doing 8 times. Add 2 or 3 each week until you work up to 15.

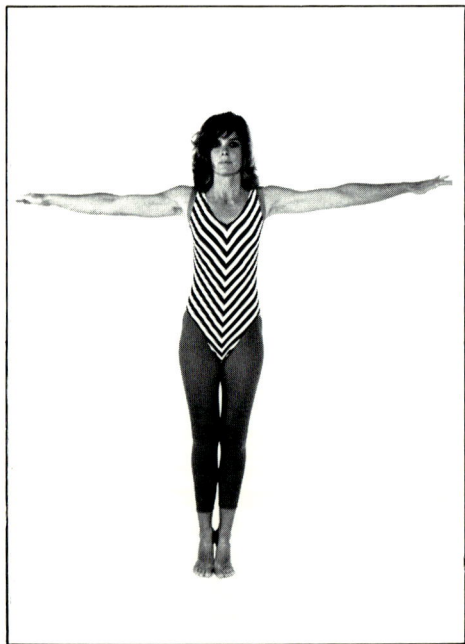

Stomach & Waistline Twist

This exercise combines twisting and stretching as another way of achieving total body involvement.

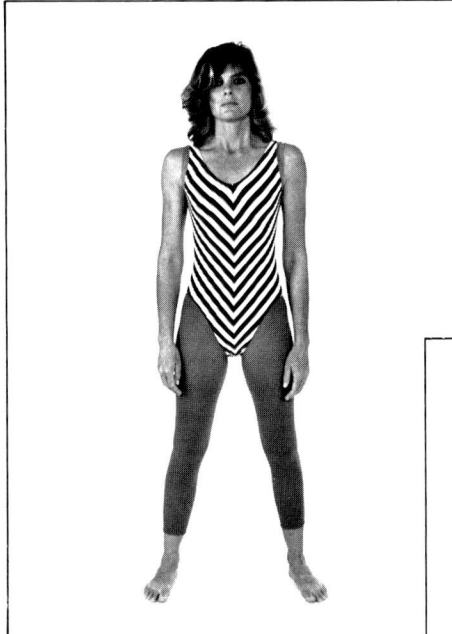

Stand straight. Body aligned, facing straight ahead with feet apart.

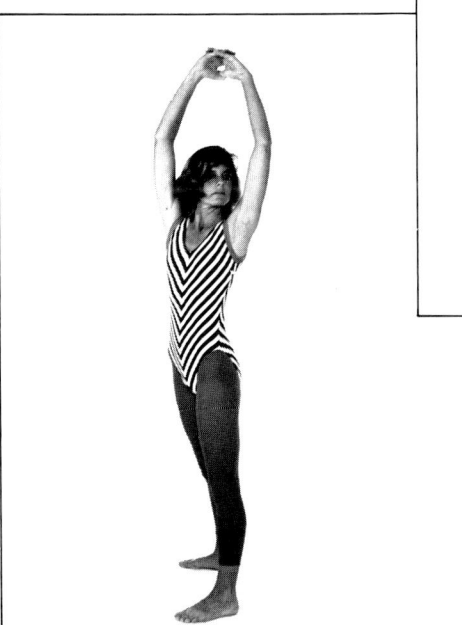

Raise your arms over your head and clasp your hands. Hips facing forward.

Twist, lifting your body up.

Bend down and touch your toes.

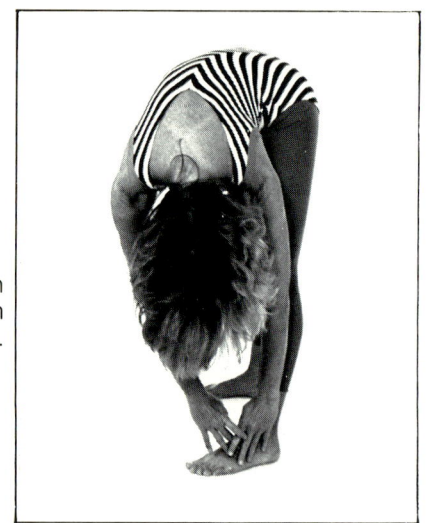

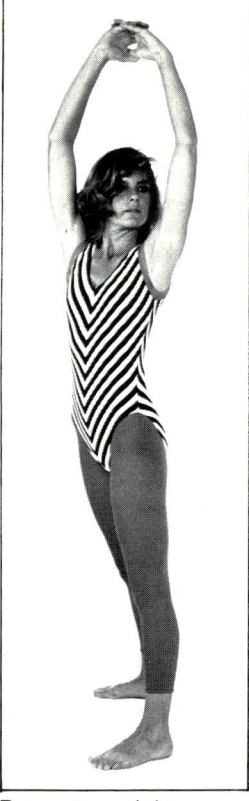

Return to upright position. Straighten.

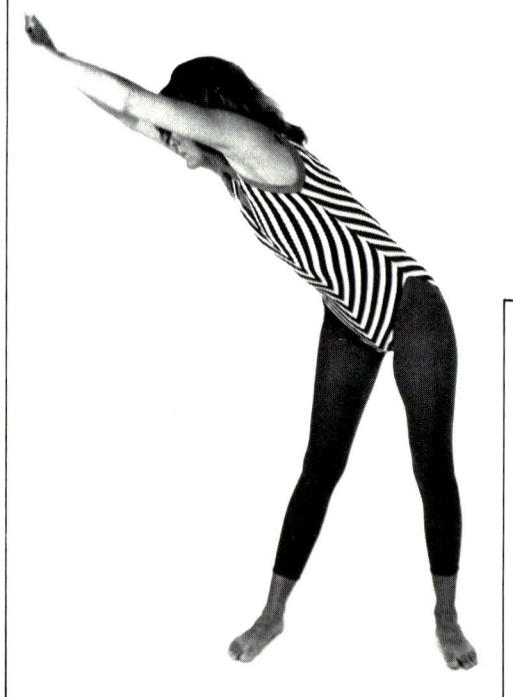

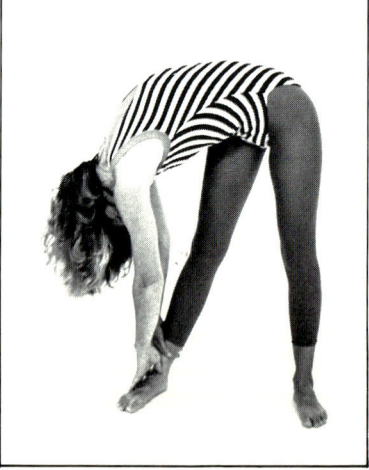

Twist and bend to repeat exercise on the other side. Begin with 3 to each side, adding 3 each week until you're doing 12 on each side.

How to Take Proper Body Measurements

Katharine demonstrates how to take these ever-so-vital statistics. You should do this once each week and record the results. See Chapter 21, on Maintenance, for detailed instructions.

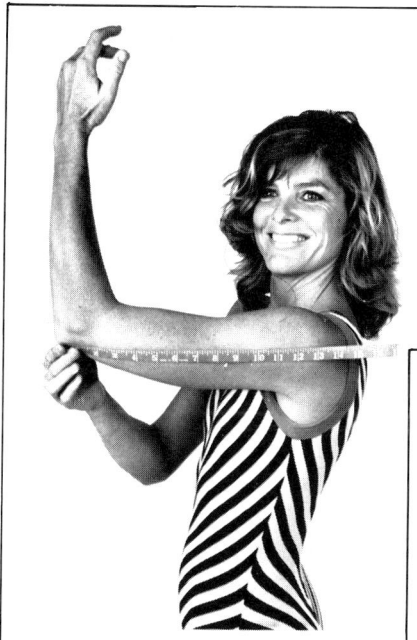

Arm measurements.

a) From elbow to largest part of arm.
b) Circumference.

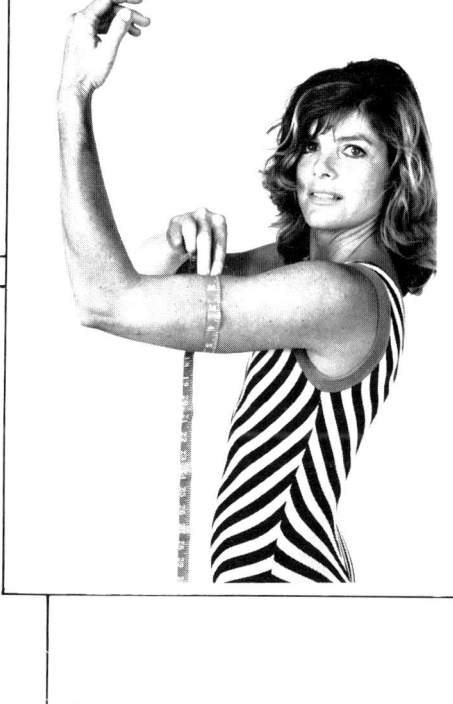

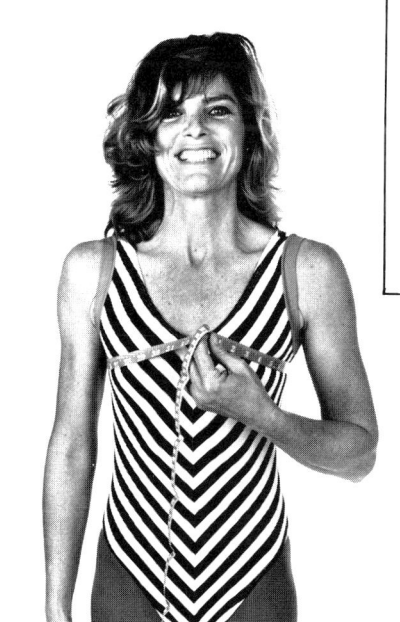

Chest measurement.

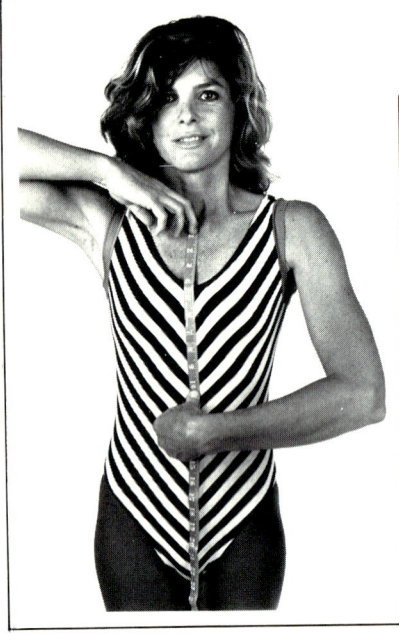

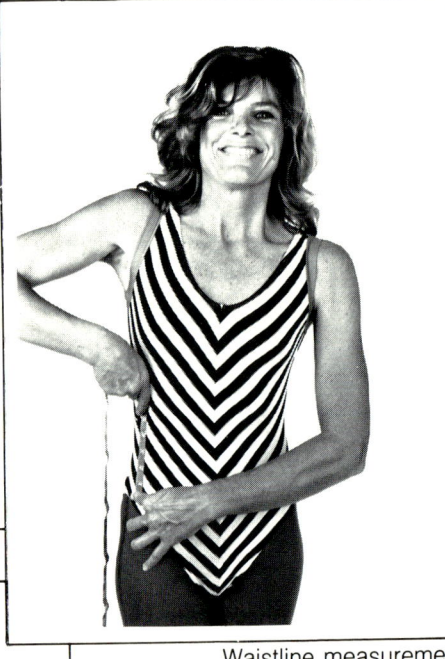

Diaphragm measurement.

Waistline measurement.

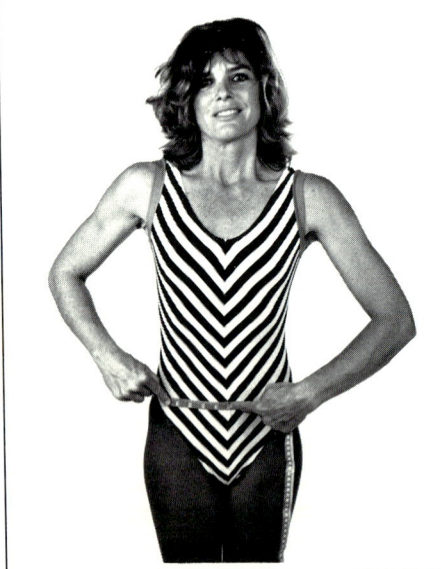

Stomach measurement.

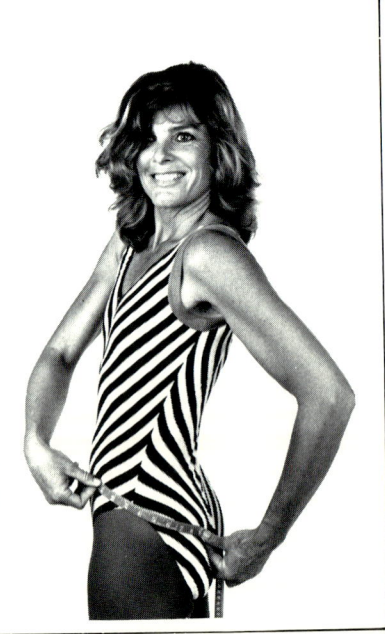

Posterior measurement.

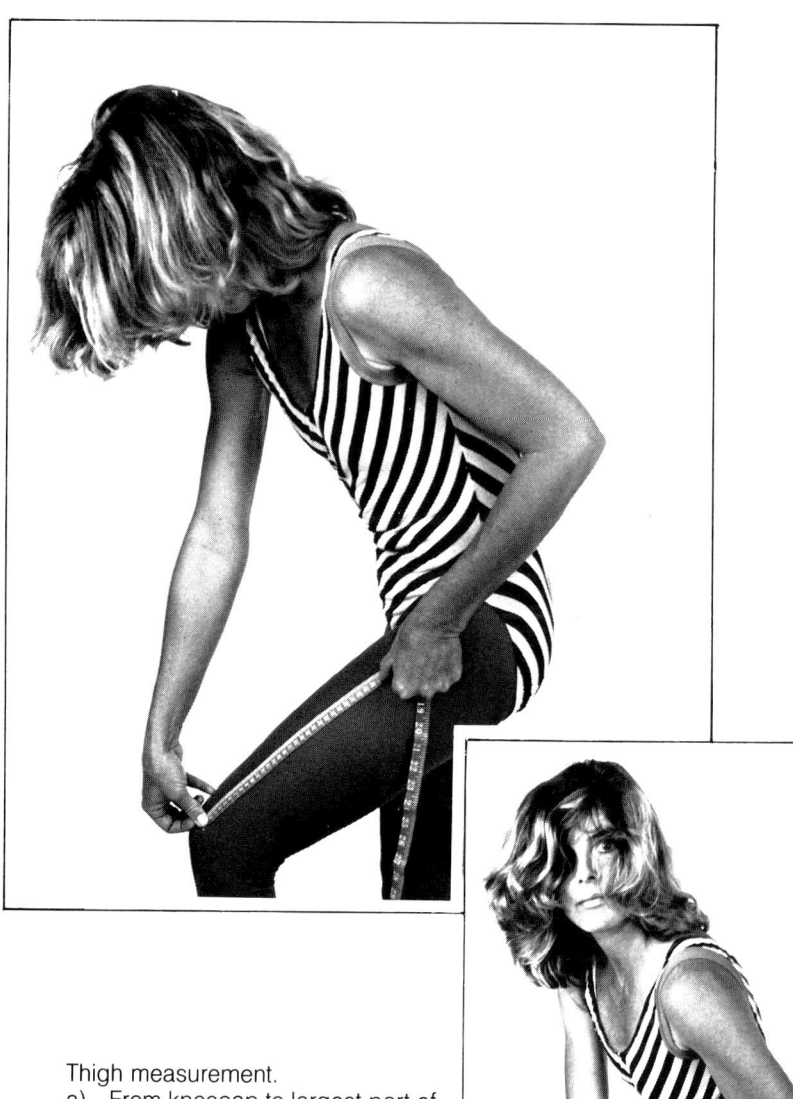

Thigh measurement.
a) From kneecap to largest part of thigh.
b) Circumference.

Dramatic Before and After Results

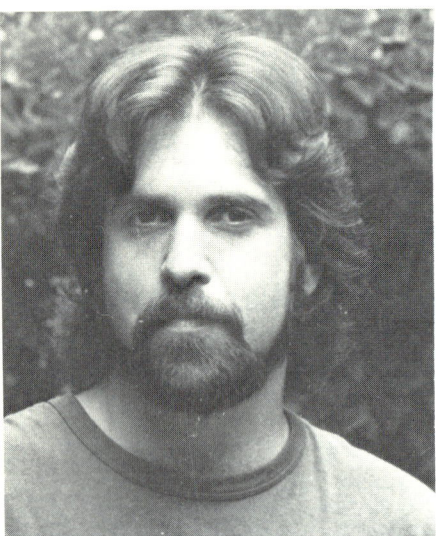

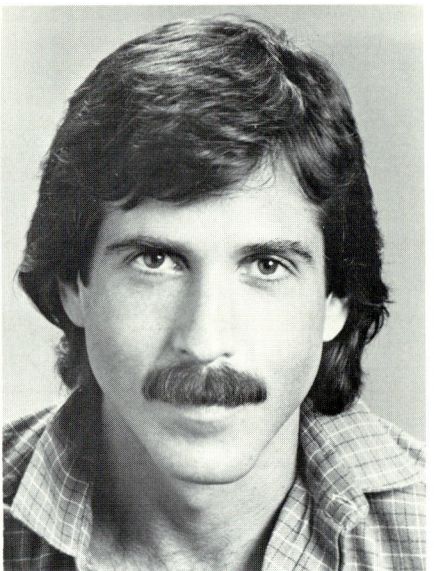

Bobby Colomby, former drummer of Blood, Sweat and Tears, came to Hermien to lose weight all over—but particularly to shape his face. Here are the results.
a) Before

b) After (photograph by Michael Maron)

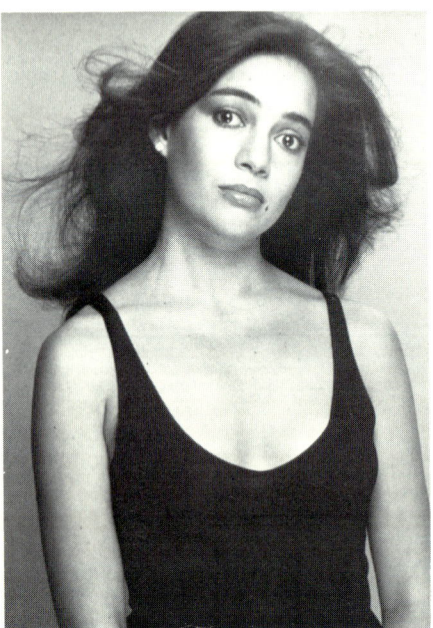

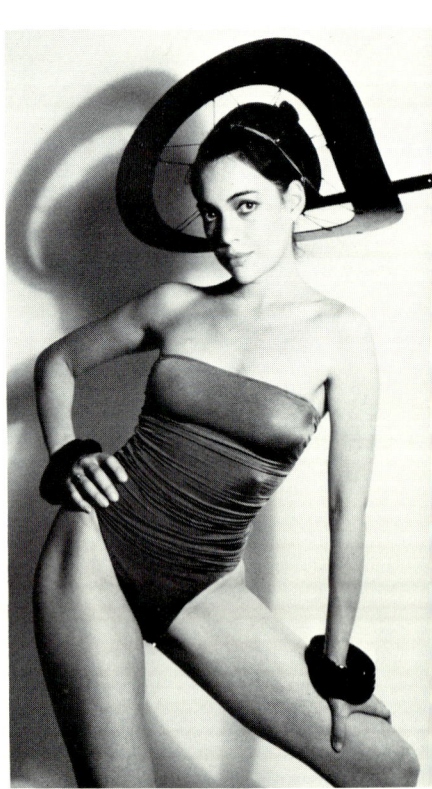

Award-winning actress Julie Carmen shaped up all over.
a) Before

b) After (photograph by Sheyla Baykal)

can even be creative with nonfat milk. Add a teaspoon of vanilla or try heating it. You'll discover that after a couple of months whole milk will taste so rich with fat that you won't want to drink it. It'll taste like pure half-and-half. Your taste buds will eventually prefer the light, fresh taste of nonfat milk. And, if you're planning to breast-feed, you'll have to increase your intake of fluids. Nonfat milk will be beneficial for both you and your infant.

Baby's Body Type

What you eat may be a deciding factor in determining your baby's shape. Scientists now believe that fat cells can develop in the fetus during the sixth month of pregnancy. That means that you, the expectant mother, can help your child be a lean ectomorph instead of a plump mesomorph or a pudgy endomorph.

Sunny Griffin, TV talk show host, came to me when she was six months pregnant. She wanted to be sure that her baby was getting the right nutrients and wanted to keep her weight within a reasonable range and didn't want to end up with unnecessary bumps and bulges. We discussed everything she'd been eating. We eliminated junk food. I warned her against eating foods containing too much sugar and fat.

Sunny followed the Spot Reducing Diet, balancing her nutrients and drinking nonfat milk. When her baby was born the pediatrician said she was the healthiest child he had ever examined. I won't pretend that Sunny's diet had everything to do with the health of her baby but I will say that the better you balance your nutrients the greater chance you'll have of having a healthy baby.

Dollars and Food Sense

Being pregnant is going to challenge your food sense and your *will power*. Temptation will lurk around every aisle in the supermarket. Waiters will swoop down with the dessert tray and say, "Oh, go on—treat yourself. You're eating for two!"

Recently two former clients met in my waiting room. They had each had a baby within the last few months and as one remarked to me, "I saw myself sitting across from me. We'd both eaten ourselves silly. Neither one of us believed you."

I have four children. I ran the emotional gamut just like everyone else. The only difference was that I forced myself to steer clear of situations I knew would put my sugar addiction to too much of a test. I knew myself well enough to know that if dessert was to be served with dinner and I was emotionally ripe for whatever sweet thing was set in front of me, I'd excuse myself and leave the table. I would walk away from temptation because that was the only way I could avoid giving myself permission. Outsmart your emotions! Use your brain!

Being pregnant means being supersensitive to everything: your environment, noise, temperature, how fabric feels, or even how the refrigerator smells. Your perspective on people will become more finely tuned. You'll become more vulnerable and self-protective in relation to other people: what they say, how they say it and even how they look at you.

Your hormones are putting your whole body through daily changes. And, as this supersensitive, self-protective mother-to-be, you may find yourself in an emotional bind from time to time.

You're out with friends and everyone's drinking but you. You feel left out. Your husband's enjoying himself but you have to say, "No, thanks," and play the martyr. You can't give yourself permission to go whole hog on dessert since you know it's not good for either you or your baby.

Naturally you're going to be frustrated. Your emotions are running high and you want something that will alter your mood. There's an echo in your head: "Oh, go on . . . a glass of wine isn't going to hurt anything . . . and I used to love potato chips . . . I'm so big now so what if I get a little bigger—"

The occasional glass of wine *probably* won't hurt you or your baby, but doctors and scientists still don't know how much or how little alcohol will have a permanently damaging effect. No one can give you personal specifics since every body is different.

One potato chip contains approximately 20 calories. Three and one-half ounces of potato chips, a medium-sized bag, contains between 550 and 575 calories. So a few handfuls will contain hundreds of fat-saturated calories. You'll be getting saddlebags to go with your expanding midriff.

Okay, you can't drink, you can't smoke, you can't take aspirin or eat junk food. What's left? How can you treat yourself without causing bumps and bulges? What can you do to reward yourself?

One of the best ways to improve both mental and physical well-being is to exercise. In some cities there are special exercise classes for expectant mothers. Check with your YWCA or local college or university. If there isn't a class in your area, you can buy a book with special exercises such as Femmy Delyser's, or a videotape. Walking and swimming are also excellent. But ask your doctor what he advises for *you*.

Exercise will help you keep your spots in check. Your muscles need toning whether you're pregnant or not. Exercise will help you relieve tension and anxiety. The calmer you feel, the easier it is to avoid bingeing. Exercise will improve your circulation and your baby's circulation. The better you feel the easier it will be for you to deal with the emotional highs and lows.

If you think of pregnancy as an athletic event, you'll be on the right track. Each day, each week, and each month bring you just that much closer to the main event. Eating properly and keeping your weight within a reasonable, healthy range will make giving birth easier on both you and your baby.

Instead of rewarding yourself with spot-making foods, reward yourself with a lasting creative endeavor: decorate the nursery, knit something for baby, sew something for yourself or baby, go on a shopping expedition or to a movie. Once the baby arrives, your activities will be severely curtailed. Make the most of your prebirth time. Go to the symphony or take a long, leisurely walk. Get out! Don't pack it in!

Plan Ahead

Since you and your baby are what you eat you might as well select the best variety of fruits and vegetables the season has to offer. Make grocery shopping fun! Take your time. Select Hit the Spot foods that you've never tried. Experiment; be creative. Keep your pantry and refrigerator stocked with plenty of things you can have. If you must stuff your face, make sure it's with something that's on the list.

Make up a number of dinners and freeze them. Many of the

recipes that feature chicken breasts are very good for this purpose. After you've had the baby, you're going to need to rest, recuperate, and feel pampered. Preparing food ahead of time will insure your dietary needs. By planning ahead you will be able to rest easier.

During your pregnancy it's important for you to eat three square meals plus a couple of snacks. Never skip a meal because you think you're gaining too much weight. Let your doctor advise you about your weight.

Eating the proper balance of nutrients should keep you regular. If you need more fiber, try three tablespoons a day of Miller's bran. Constipation is most common when there is a marked imbalance in one's diet. Being pregnant and bogged down is to be avoided at all costs.

Television commercials proclaim the great virtues of Alka-Seltzer. It may be a wonderful solution for indigestion when you're not pregnant, but when you are, doctors and scientists recommend avoiding it. You should check with your doctor before taking *any* medication. Indigestion is usually brought on by overeating or by eating what I call the exotic heart-burners: pastrami, curry, a dish loaded with garlic. Use your food sense.

One of the great rewards of eating sensibly is that after you've given birth your body will be able to return to its prepregnant weight more quickly and easily.

Biggest Offenders in Pregnancy

If you overeat highly fatted foods beyond your daily needs, you not only build fat cells in your child at six months but you also fill up the fat cells in your legs and posterior. Here are the biggest offenders to posterior, hips, saddlebags, knees:

avocados
butter
chips of any kind
chocolate
duck
fat on any meat
French fries
highly fatted meats
ice cream
margarine
nuts
olives
pastry
salami, pastrami, corned beef
sour cream
whipping cream

And for waistline, stomach, upper hips, back, arms and face:

cookies high in sugar	pie
crackers	potato—too much
donuts	pretzels
hard candy	regular chewing gum
jam	rice—too much
Jell-O	soft drinks with sugar
jelly, honey, and sugar	sweet and sour anything
pasta	bread—too much

Too much carbohydrate also makes you retain water.

18

NURSING

Never diet to lose weight when you're breast-feeding. After you've given birth, don't be surprised if you still look six months pregnant. Very few mothers can fit into their prepregnant wardrobe within months of the blessed event.

Naturally, your abdomen is going to be prominent, and even with exercise your waistline won't automatically shrink to its former size. These spots are expected to be exaggerated. It's the other spots—arms, back, backside, legs—that may have gotten out of proportion when you were pregnant.

Often it's not until after one has given birth that the true nature of her shape comes into sharp focus. If you have lumps and bumps where you used to have them or where you never had them before, remember two things: you gained weight over a nine-month period and now the only safe and sensible way to lose it is *slowly,* over a period of months. Going on a crash diet does not allow your body to repair itself. Your body has gone through enormous changes and it needs plenty of time to readjust. Proper nutrition is one of your most important healing devices.

Now is not the time to diet to lose weight. It is, however, a time when you can lose unattractive spots. Read the chapter that corresponds to the spot you wish to eliminate. That will give you an understanding about the foods that caused you to gain weight in that specific area.

Now, about all you can do with your old clothes is look at them. You feel fat, out of proportion, even ugly. You want to lose weight as quickly as possible but *you should not jeopardize your or your infant's health by going on a crash diet.* Cutting back too much, not getting enough nutritional fuel, will make you weak because it deprives you of necessary nutrients. When you go on a crash diet all you get is a hollow, gaunt face—your top half may shrink a little, you may lose a few pounds, but your body's not going to lose weight *evenly.* Your spots will be even more pronounced. Balancing your nutrients is essential to nursing as well as to eliminating lumps and bumps. Eating properly will help you lose weight evenly and just by not eating junk you'll lose a few pounds.

Your baby draws from you so it's your responsibility to maintain all the nutrients both of you need. Nursing takes more out of you than pregnancy. It's even more nutritionally demanding—as the baby grows you must produce more milk. And if your infant is to gain weight and grow healthy, he's going to need the right balance of nutrients. Be sure to check with your doctor for the vitamin you should take.

The nursing mother needs:

50 percent more calcium and vitamin A;
40 percent more protein and riboflavin;
33 percent more vitamin C and thiamine;
25 percent more calories than a nonpregnant mother.

Drink eight glasses of fluid a day; make six of them vitamin A- and D-fortified nonfat milk if you can. Drink a lot of water—bottled if your tap water is high in pollutants. Drink coffee, tea, or diet drinks in moderation.

When Linda Lane had her baby she read the hospital pamphlets on breast-feeding. They emphasized drinking lots of liquids. Juice was included on the list. She ordered orange juice and apple juice with her dinner, grapefruit juice with breakfast, and more apple juice with lunch. She thought she was getting the fluid she needed, plus a little extra energy from the fruit. She got more than she bargained for.

"I was exhausted and I thought I needed the extra sugar in juice to keep me going. Breast-feeding a newborn baby every two hours is pretty draining—figuratively and literally. What I didn't realize was that all the sugar and acid in the juice were going through me, into my milk and into my baby. I didn't know what to do when Lucy started screaming. She was fussy and colicky. I told Hermien the symptoms and she asked what I was eating and drinking. When I told her about the juice in the hospital and loads of apple juice when I got home, she told me to stop drinking it immediately. She said that instead I should drink plenty of water and that I should *eat* my allotted three pieces of fruit a day. I went back on the Spot Reducing Diet, adding six glasses of nonfat milk a day. I ordered bottled water delivered to my house. I went back to measuring everything. If I had shredded wheat for breakfast I measured half a cup. If I had salad for lunch I measured the vegetables and weighed my protein out. I didn't leave anything to the imagination. I found I had more energy, and Lucy no longer suffered from the excess sugar and acid I had been overloading her with.

"Slowly, but dramatically, my spots melted away. My husband was the most amazed. He'd been skeptical from the start. It took about two to three months to lose and redistribute the weight. The more religiously I followed Hermien's program the faster my body reproportioned itself. I also continued taking my prenatal vitamins and exercising for a few minutes every day."

From Shapeless to Shapely

Every new mother would like to go from shapeless to shapely as quickly as possible. And fortunately, Mother Nature designed breast-feeding as a reciprocal arrangement.

Human milk is the best-balanced, most easily digestible food for a human baby. Besides providing all the nutrients your baby needs, it contains antibodies and immunity factors to the illnesses you've had—measles and mumps, for example—or been immunized against. This has nothing to do with the immunizations your child will receive from the pediatrician.

Dr. Steven Shapiro, a Los Angeles pediatrician, says, "Breast-fed babies are generally healthier than bottle-fed babies in the first few years of life." He recommends nursing for the first eight months. "But if you breast-feed for a month, it's better than not doing it at all. Most women in this practice breast-feed for the first eight months. Then they generally wean the baby onto a cup."

When bab nurses, his suckling action signals your organs that it's time to go back in place. Your pituitary gland releases a hormone called *oxytocin* that makes your uterus contract. Those contractions help push waste down and out while helping the uterus to shrink back to normal. Oxytocin does several things. It causes your milk to be forced through your milk ducts and then into pools beneath the areols. Oxytocin is what's responsible for making your milk available to baby. It's also released during childbirth and during orgasm.

The more you nurse, the more milk you'll produce. The longer you nurse, eating properly, the better shape you'll be in. And the better you balance your nutrients, the more quickly your spots will disappear.

Some of the fat your body stored when you were pregnant was nature's way of preparing you for the demands of nursing. If the body is getting everything it needs it won't have to store fat for a potential emergency. Weight will come off naturally.

Exercise is the other key to going from shapeless to shapely. Your muscles are stretched. Your bones had to shift and so did your organs. Exercise gets your circulation going, it gives you more energy and it tones your tired muscles. You can exercise at home or, in some cities, there are recovery classes to which mothers can bring their babies. I've seen amazing results with women who've combined the Spot Reducing Diet with an exercise program soon after giving birth. Within a couple of months most of them are back to their prepregnant shapes.

Eating for Two

Everything about a new baby is *new*. His stomach and digestive tract must *learn* to function.

When you were pregnant, if you ate something that gave you indigestion, only you suffered. Now, if you eat something that gives your baby an acid stomach, a lot of gas, or any variation on that unpleasant theme, both you and your baby will suffer.

Your milk is composed of everything you eat and drink. Baby may not like *curried* milk. Raw onions or garlic might give him gas.

Keep thinking moderation. *Try a little* and if all goes well, try a little more. Don't think that because you've always eaten highly spiced food, your newborn is ready for it. As the weeks and then the months pass you will be able to add more and more foods to your diet.

Many of my clients have been told that drinking beer or wine makes breast-feeding easier. That's an old wives' tale. A glass of wine may help a nervous mother relax but it's certainly not necessary to the act of nursing. The *occasional* glass of wine is fine.

As Linda learned, beer can be very fattening. "I was told that drinking imported beer helped calm you down and increase your milk supply. My husband gave me German beer because it was rich and yeasty. I developed a real taste for it. I mentioned what I was doing to Hermien and she asked me if my stomach was going down. It told her it wasn't and she told me to stop drinking beer and it would.

"I'd given myself permission to drink beer because it relaxed me and it did taste good. But, once again, Hermien was right. After I gave it up my stomach went down noticeably."

Create a peaceful environment when you're nursing. Baby's emotional life is tied directly to you. If you get upset, baby will sense your uneasy feelings and he'll get upset too. Your being upset is one of the reasons babies get fussy and colicky. Stress can cause you to decrease your milk supply. Stay calm. Take the phone off the hook. Drink six glasses of vitamin A- and D-fortified nonfat milk every day—the calcium will help keep both you and your infant calm. Drink plenty of water and everything else in moderation.

Increasing Your Milk Supply

The key ingredient in increasing your milk supply is brewer's yeast—and you don't have to drink beer to get it. You can take it in less fattening ways that will benefit you more.

Brewer's yeast has a strange, unpleasant taste at first, but don't let that dissuade you. If you need to increase your milk supply, a few days of brewer's yeast should do the trick. The following recipe, which you should have once a day, will help you stay on the Spot Reducing Diet while enhancing your diet with brewer's yeast. After a few days you may even grow to like the unusual taste. And once you've increased your milk supply you can stop taking it.

BREWER'S YEAST FEAST

1 large orange, peeled
1 T. brewer's yeast
3 ice cubes, crushed
¼ cup vitamin A- and D-fortified nonfat milk
1 T. specially prepared peanut butter (optional)

Place crushed ice in a blender or food processor and add the peeled orange sections. Turn the motor on. When the orange is juiced, add the other ingredients and whip into a frothy, refreshing drink. The taste of brewer's yeast will be disguised and you should find yourself with a burst of energy and an increase in your milk supply.

Don't Overfeed Baby

There are many schools of thought on bringing up baby. One of them suggests that when baby cries he wants to be fed, changed, or cuddled. Try not to feed more than every two hours. If you feed *on demand,* as some call it, you may be giving both you and your baby a problem.

It takes about two hours for each meal to digest. If baby's crying about something else—boredom, discomfort, gas, hiccups—and you think you can quiet him by another feeding, all you're doing is adding fuel to the fire. If baby has a stomach ache, another meal may make it more painful.

As the baby gets older, increase the time between feedings. Your infant should go for three hours, then four hours between feedings. And if your milk is satisfying baby, by the time he's two months old he might sleep for a six- to eight-hour stretch. It takes about three months before an infant's digestive tract is in good working order, before you can kiss colic good-bye.

If you have questions about nursing, there are a number of good books on the subject. It's wise to take a course if you're a first-time mother. Breast-feeding, contrary to some opinions, does not always come naturally.

Some babies are born with an urge to latch on and suck. Others, often called tongue-suckers because they prefer playing to nursing, must be positioned, repositioned, talked to, cajoled, and even tricked into latching on and sucking. If you can stick with it, your baby will become a good eater. Remember: the longer you nurse the better shape you'll be in.

One excellent source of information is:

> La Leche League
> 9616 Minneapolis Avenue
> Franklin Park, IL 60131

Check your local telephone directory for a branch of the La Leche League near you. It is a nonprofit organization made up of supportive mothers who can direct you to good sources of material, classes, or even personal assistance.

Breast-feeding has many built-in advantages in today's nonstop world. The food is always handy, always the right temperature, bacteria-free, and loaded with antibodies and immunity factors. It's the best way to give your child both the physical and emotional nourishment he or she needs. If you become ill while breast-feeding, check with your physician immediately.

As you follow the Spot Reducing Diet, adding your nonfat milk, your body will slowly and naturally return to its former shape. You won't feel hungry or deprived.

The most enjoyable part of nursing is the bonding process that takes place between you and your child. As your child breast-feeds, stimulating you to produce more milk, you will become the person who gives him a sense of continuity and security. Bonding is a way of providing emotional nourishment as well as physical nourishment. It is a wonderful reciprocal arrangement.

19

OVERWEIGHT CHILDREN AND TEENAGERS

There are two types of overweight children and teenagers—the ones who need to trim a spot here or there and the ones who have so many spots they need to reduce all over.

For individual spots, read the chapter that corresponds to the areas you're interested in trimming. The same balance of protein, fat, and carbohydrate that works for adults works for children and teenagers.

Since both children and teenagers are still growing, *add one quart of vitamin A- and D-fortified nonfat milk to the daily program*. I also recommend including a multivitamin/mineral. Ask your pediatrician which one to take.

Children

Children can be overweight because they eat too much at home or somewhere else. They may be given a good, balanced lunch which they trade at school for candy and chips. Whatever the cause, changing the overweight result is going to take a lot of help and cooperation from everyone involved.

Dr. Steven Shapiro believes that the key to children's changing their eating habits and losing weight is motivation. "You find with adolescents," he says, "that generally if they're motivated they will lose weight. However, if you see an obese child ten or eleven years old in your office and you recommend some nutritional counseling, if the child isn't motivated and the parents aren't motivated it's a total failure. It's a very rough situation in that overweight children and teenagers tend to have poor body images. They tend to have less self-esteem and it goes on and on into adulthood."

In my experience the best way to motivate overweight children is to help them understand the relationship between what they eat and, if they overeat, where it goes on the body: drawing a clear equation between eating too much carbohydrate—hard candy, soft drinks, too much bread, cookies, and too much fruit—and having a big stomach, a fat back, big arms, and a round face. Or to tell them about being a fat addict and eating foods loaded with visible and invisible fat: how bacon and fried eggs, toast slathered with butter, lots of cheese, ice cream, milk shakes, yogurt, tuna packed in oil with mayonnaise, and chocolate will give one a broad behind and big legs.

Then there's the child who eats too much protein—meat, nuts, cheese, fish, poultry, and dairy products—who gets big and seemingly muscular all over. When this child hits the spot he shrinks evenly all over. This is especially nice for girls, because losing weight all over makes them look as well as feel more feminine.

Losing weight and changing eating habits is hard work, so do your best to make it fun. Make it into a game so that you can repeat the information as many times as it takes to give your child a positive feeling for what he or she is doing. Helping your child now may do a lifetime of good.

One of my most challenging clients was eight-year-old, 200-pound Bill. He didn't like regular milk, so he drank gallons of half-and-half. He ate butter by the spoonful and huge amounts of protein until his behind and legs were so big that his parents had to have his pants specially made. He ate so much candy that he looked like an inflated clown—his stomach hung over his pants and his face was moon-shaped.

When Bill started with me I got his attention by telling him that his body was his hotel. Pointing at an anatomical illustration I said, "That's where Mary Gallbladder lives. There's John Liver and that's where Ozzie Intestine lives. When you give them good service they're happy to live in your hotel. In fact, they'll even help you. They'll make you feel great! You'll feel lighter and you'll have more energy. But when you clog up the corridors," I said, pointing at the intestine, "with too much food, you're giving them bad service. Bad service in your hotel makes them uncomfortable and angry because they have to work harder. They want to move out but they can't. They're stuck, so they rebel. They give you gas, they make you tired, they may even get so angry they give you a stomach ache. So, brother," I concluded, "you just better clean up your corridors!"

Bill looked at me and without saying another word stood up and marched out of my office. I didn't know if I was ever going to see him again.

Four days later I got a call. "Hermien, this is Bill. I cleaned up my corridors!" He hung up. He'd gotten the message and with the help of his family he was ready to hit all his spots.

The first spot to go down was his stomach. He started developing a waistline and then he started losing in his shoulders and arms. After two months on the Spot Reducing Diet (plus one quart of vitamin A- and D-fortified nonfat milk a day and a multivitamin/mineral) he was smaller all over. What Bill had lost in weight he'd gained in confidence. He was finally able to participate in school sports and to feel like one of the gang. Over a six-month period he lost 80 pounds. He is now nine years old and even though he's still careful to follow the program he has a balanced body.

Bill's mother played a major role in helping him lose weight. She made the Spot Reducing Diet a way of life for the whole family. Those who didn't need to lose weight added extra protein or whatever they wanted while Bill kept to the Master Plan. That made the youngster feel like an insider instead of an obese outsider.

The whole family learned something about good nutrition because Bill made it a point to tell them which foods were protein, fat, and carbohydrate. The more he learned the more anxious he was to learn more and to stick with the program. While they used to say, "Hey, Fatty, don't eat that! It'll make you fatter!" They now said, "Gosh, how can you have so much will power?"

Advice to Parents

1. *Help your child make a list of everything he's eaten each day.* Children, like adults, can suffer from hand-to-mouth disease. They

eat things without even realizing it—until they write *everything* down.

2. *Never give them permission because you want their love.* Never make food a reward. Never give an overweight child permission to eat ice cream and cake unless it's a special occasion. It may bring on a momentary smile but in the long run your child will like you far more for helping him or her form good, balanced eating habits.

3. *Make grocery shopping a group effort.* Help your child understand which foods fall into the protein, fat, and carbohydrate categories. The better informed your child is the better his or her chances of losing weight and maintaining a well-proportioned shape afterward.

4. *Always have food available that is on the Spot Reducing Diet.*

5. *Give your child his own food space.* A shelf in the refrigerator and a special space in the pantry will help your child be a successful dieter.

6. *Be supportive!* Reward your child with something other than food when a celebration is in order. When you notice spots disappearing, compliment her. Make eating properly something that is rewarded not only by a shapely difference but by your continuing encouragement.

7. *Always teach—never preach!* Telling a child not to eat something because it'll make him fat will make him angry. Telling a child that eating a box of chocolate candy will give her a big behind and big legs may make her think twice before making her spots bigger.

8. Add one quart of vitamin A- and D-fortified nonfat milk to the daily spot reducing program.

9. Ask your pediatrican to recommend a multivitamin/mineral for your child.

To Teenagers: About Teen Spots

The shape of your body will depend on two major factors: the kind of food you've grown up with and your food habits. Either one or both of these elements must be recognized before a permanent change can take place.

You may come from a family in which cooking with butter and oil is as natural as watching TV. Soul food is delicious but very high in fat. If you've been raised on soul food and fried food, the chances are you have a big behind and saddlebags. That goes for both boys and girls. You may come from an all-American apple-pie-loving junk-food family. Breakfast may start with Hostess Twinkies, fried pancakes, syrup, bacon, and hot chocolate; lunch might be a cheeseburger, French fries and a Coke; your afternoon snack might be a candy bar and for dinner the family might share a big everything-on-it pizza! Then again, you may come from an *organic* family in which everything purports to be *good for you*. You may eat loads of cheese, drink cartons of whole milk and Kefir. You may eat too much yogurt and too much tofu and trail mix by the handful. You may simply eat too much and as a result be big all over.

Start by writing down everything you eat or drink as soon as possible. Getting in touch with your true food habits is different from *thinking* you eat a certain way. Most of my teenaged clients have little or no idea what they really eat until they are forced to list everything that goes into their mouths. A lot of overweight people block out what they don't want to acknowledge. So in order to come to grips with what caused your spots, confront yourself with everything you eat and drink every day. And, if you're honest with yourself, if you want something but you don't want to write it down because you know it's loaded with sugar or fat or it's more than your daily allowance, you simply must not eat it. And if you know yourself well enough to know that you can't be honest, realize that you will not be a successful dieter. It takes a balanced diet to have a balanced shape.

If you're out of balance—if you have ugly spots—the time when you're a teenager is the time to lose them. As you refine your lumps and bumps your youthful skin will tighten up because it has a wonderful elasticity that one loses as one gets older. Of course, exercise helps too.

Talk yourself into being patient. Programs don't work for most teenagers because they are looking for magic. If the scale is your god, if the needle doesn't go down every day and you get frustrated and binge, you will set your life's course as a yoyoer. Going from deprivation to rewarding yourself with the wrong food will make your spots even worse.

The Spot Reducing Diet is not a fad diet. It is a way of life. It's a way of changing your eating habits so that you can reshape your body *without suffering* (you won't go hungry) and learn how to keep it in perfect proportion for the rest of your life.

When you start the program you must stick with it for a least three weeks. No cheating! I'm giving you the tools with which you and you alone can reshape your body. Your color will improve, your complexion will be clear, or at least less likely to get pimples; even your hair will have a healthier shine. Remember, *you are your own magic*. You didn't get yourself out of proportion in a week. The more slowly you lose and redistribute your weight, the better the odds are of your stabilizing your weight and maintaining your attractive new shape.

Eat everything every day, or you won't see the balance I'm talking about. Don't cut down on anything listed in the Master Plan because you think you'll lose spots faster. If you don't like something on one of the daily menus, make a switch, using the substitution lists. You can also make your own menu, using the Master Plan as a guide.

Be Patient!

The reason my overweight teenagers succeed is that they stick to the program until the dramatic change occurs. Jamie Gross came to me when she was 16. She was a darling girl with a pear shape—petite, and muscular from playing five hours of sports every day. I told her that her body could be perfectly proportioned. She didn't have to have big legs if she'd be patient and do everything I told her to do.

She was skeptical. She started crying when I told her all the things I wanted her to eat. "I can't do that," she said. "I'll gain weight. That's more than I've ever eaten! No way!"

"Jamie," I said, "just trust me and give me two weeks. If it doesn't work you can go back to starving yourself."

"At the time I went to Hermien," Jamie admits, "I was refusing to eat. She believed that I was getting anorexia and she wouldn't have anything to do with me unless I promised that I wasn't and that I would give her two weeks. If it didn't work her way, she told me I could go back to doing it my way. In the beginning she wanted me to gain three pounds to get my metabolism back up and then, all of a sudden, she said I would shrink. And I did. I shrank right in front of everyone's eyes. In a month I was down to where I wanted to be. And I've stayed there.

"I used to go for candy—I just loved candy," she continues. "It gave me energy before sports. Now I just eat an orange and a Laughing Cow Green Label cheese wedge. I never eat candy anymore but now I could if I wanted because I know I'd never binge out. But it took me a year of staying away from it—I couldn't go near it because I knew if I did I'd eat the whole thing. I can live without sugar now. In the beginning I went through the worst sugar withdrawal. I just slept all day. I couldn't get out of bed. You don't realize how much sugar you eat—it's incredible. So I was just sleeping all day. That's why I won't eat sugar again. I don't have to have a dependence on it."

Sugar Blues

Sugar withdrawal is rough for anyone of any age. It seems especially difficult for teenagers because sweets seem to be part of growing up. Sweet-sixteen parties, birthday parties, having a Coke at a football game and a box of chocolate-covered raisins at the movies. If sugar is your thing, be prepared to experience withdrawal symptoms. (See Sugar Withdrawal, p. 25.)

Peer Pressure

"I'm on a diet" goes down about as well as cold glue. Diet is a four-letter word; those who aren't on one will try to push off those who are. It's popular to have a perfectly proportioned body but it isn't popular to refuse food and drink.

Jamie Gross has some excellent advice for overcoming peer pressure. It's always going to be there, because it's part of growing up, but there are ways to be part of the gang without eating and drinking spot-producing foods.

Jamie suggests, "It's a lot easier to say, 'I don't like French fries even if you do.' If you are dieting, don't tell anyone, because automatically they take notice of you. I always say, 'How can you eat that greasy thing?' About French fries: if you say you can't eat them because you don't like them rather than because they're fattening, they can't put pressure on you. I use the excuse that I have a really fragile stomach. That's the one I always use because your friends aren't going to want to make you sick and suffer."

Once you balance your nutrients you balance your body, and you become more emotionally centered. When everybody starts *partying*, which often translates to drinking wine, beer, or hard liquor or smoking dope, if you're in control of your emotions it's so much easier to participate in the social activities without partaking of the spot-producing, mind-altering substances. Alcoholic beverages will give you a paunchy stomach and a puffy face, and will make you bloated. Marijuana gives people the munchies, or hand-to-mouth disease. If you're not thinking clearly, it's all too easy to stuff your face with whatever's handy: chips, ice cream, candy. You lose your food sense and you add lumps and bumps to your body.

When asked how Jamie handles drinking and peer pressure she said, "Drinking to me is a waste of calories. The biggest waste of calories. I could be having three oranges instead of a drink. That's the way I look at it. I'd rather have something I enjoy than a drink with my friends. When you look sensational you don't have to worry about your peers pushing you off your diet. The way I look," she says, smiling with a well deserved sense of confidence, "takes the place of having to get drunk or do dope, because people tend to follow me. It's easy when I go out to eat. I never have a problem in a restaurant. There are so many things you can order, because the Spot Reducing Diet's not a diet. It's just good nutrition."

If you can be relaxed about changing your eating habits, and *refuse to be intimidated by peer pressure*, you will be able to keep pace with your friends and still hit your spots. Remember, if you join your friends at the pizza parlor and go along with the gang by eating pizza, you're sabotaging yourself. If you're going to trim spots from the waist down, the oil in a slice of pizza can set you back about a month.

You have to give it up only until you're finished—then I can teach you how to eat it.

Hints for Hitting the Spot

1. *Don't make the scale your god*. Teenagers seem to let the scale dictate when they start a diet; if they don't see the needle on the

scale going down every day they stop the program. Weigh yourself by all means, but don't let the scale push you off the program. If the scale is an obstacle, weigh yourself once a week. Ironically, when you follow the program exactly, when the scale doesn't go down is the time when your body is changing shape—losing spots.

2. *Make sure you write down everything you eat and drink every day for at least three weeks.*

3. *Ask your mother to help you.* Sit down with your mother and explain that the Spot Reducing Diet is a nutritionally balanced diet that will benefit the whole family. The recipes I've given you are delicious, low in calories, and fun to make. If you have leftovers you can freeze them. If you have the foods you are supposed to eat available you will successfully hit your spot.

4. *Make a grocery list.* To make sure you have plenty of Spot Reducing Diet choices, be sure to make a grocery list. Whether you accompany your mother to the market or you go alone, if you have a list you will be sure to get everything you need. Always plan ahead!

5. *Use a button bag.* If you find it difficult to get all your vegetables every day, make a *button bag* containing any raw vegetables you can cut into coin-shaped pieces: carrots, cucumber, zucchini, whole string beans, cauliflower or broccoli flowerets, and whole cherry tomatoes; take it with you everyplace you go. This is especially useful when you're studying.

6. *Be creative!* As long as you have two meals a day—lunch and dinner—I don't care if you change or omit menus *as long as you have all of the requirements listed on the Master Plan every day.* You can have a sandwich before bed, or half a frozen banana with specially prepared peanut butter.

7. *Use psychology.* Avoid saying, "I can't eat it, I'm on a diet." It's like sending up a red flag. It's much easier to say, "I don't eat sugar," or "I can't eat fried foods—they upset my stomach," or "I don't like candied yams," or "I don't like regular soft drinks, they're too sweet."

8. *What to do with negative energy.* When you're under pressure you build up a kind of negative energy that you just can't seem to get rid of. It's easy to push it down with food. I find that the best solution is *exercise.* Turn on your radio or stereo and dance! Do something physically active. When you're finished, know that you

can have a Spot Reducing Diet snack. This is one reason I've planned a bedtime snack on each of the daily menus.

9. *Don't yoyo!* Don't go from deprivation to reward. Never starve yourself and then go on an eating binge so that you can starve yourself again. Break that vicious circle now!

10. Never eat something because *it's there!*

11. *Plan a reward for the time when you have successfully hit your spot!* Promise yourself a new pair of jeans or a weekend skiing. Make it something you really want, so that when you're tempted or being pressured by your peers you'll have something to help you stick with the program. And when you've trimmed your spot or spots, your well balanced body will be your greatest reward. Stick with the program for at least three weeks.

EXERCISES

20

RON FLETCHER'S EXERCISE GUIDE

Ron Fletcher is considered one of the leading exercise experts in America. He has created these simple exercises—for exclusive use with the Spot Reducing Diet—so that everyone, whether athletically inclined or not, will be able to do them successfully, and enjoy them too! Fletcher believes that we must become more conscious of the total mind, body, breath machine. "It isn't enough to fling your arms about or to dangle your legs and kick to the side a dozen times. When you exercise you must involve your whole body. That means the breathing apparatus as well."

Ron believes that knowing how your body is connected—being aware of which muscle groups are performing their various functions—will help you to properly align yourself, thereby making the toning, strengthening, and body-shaping benefits more effective. "No matter what you do," Ron says, "it's only as good as your total concentration. Pay attention to body alignment!"

Whole-Body Toner

The Whole-Body Toner involves exactly what its name implies: feet, legs, posterior, stomach, spine, and on up to the neck and the top of the head. Think of a string extending up from the back of your head pulling you upward.

1. *Standing straight, ankles touching, knees together— lift your toes.* If your body is in alignment your feet will form what Ron calls a pair of triangular bases. If you are not standing correctly, the chances are that you will lose your balance.

    It is important to make each move with total attention if you are going to work all of your muscles to the optimum.
2. *Flatten your toes and with ankles and knees together lengthen your body upward.* You should be able to feel the muscles above the knees contracting. Stand in front of a mirror so that you can make sure your body is properly aligned.
3. *Concentrate on the low abdominal muscles.* Think of pulling your stomach in, using the low band of muscles located directly above the pelvic bone and connecting around the back to the muscles beneath the cheeks. These are the posterior muscles that *lift* the buttocks.
4. *Lengthen the body upward,* allowing as much space as possible between the bottom rib and your hip bone.

    This is what Ron calls an antigravity action. Your body is stretching against gravity and even though it doesn't seem like a strenuous, energy-consuming exercise, all of your muscles are working. Watch your shoulders—don't raise them!
5. *Lift sternum (chestbone) upward* so that your neck will lengthen. Lift up! Do not push out. Watch your alignment. Make sure that your head is pulled back and in alignment. Think of the top of the back of your head as the end of the spine. Think of lengthening the spine as if you are letting air between the vertebrae.
6. *Extend your arms up and out to your sides, parallel to the floor.*
7. *Make a fist and take a deep breath.*
8. *Contract your buttocks. Be careful not to raise your shoulders. Raise your eyebrows.*
9. *Release—* Breathe out, relax your hands, relax your buttocks and begin again. Repeat this exercise for ten minutes twice a day.

    When you are contracting muscles you are toning them. This exercise will be beneficial for your whole body. If you have time to do only one exercise, Ron recommends the Whole-Body Toner. He believes that it sets up a *muscle memory*—all of your muscles are being toned, everything is being integrated.

    You can even tone your muscles while you're sitting in your car, idling at a traffic light. Contract your buttocks and release, contract and release. For once you'll be able to use heavy traffic to your advantage!

Ron's Body-Lift Exercise

Standing tall, your body lengthened and aligned as in the Whole-Body Toner:
1. Contract buttocks muscles.
2. Lift up on your toes, keeping your ankles together.
3. Extend your arms to the side, parallel with the floor. (Be sure that you are balancing over the center toes. Do not roll to the outside of your feet.)
4. Lift up and come down. Lift up and take a deep breath. Slowly let it out on your way down. Begin by doing the Body Lift eight times. Add two or three each week until you are doing fifteen a day.

A few exercises done slowly use more energy than you might think, and there is more total body/mind involvement. According to Ron Fletcher, it is better to do a few minutes of slow and careful body work with total concentration than a prolonged series of mechanical kicks and twists with no thought involved.

Ron's Stomach and Waistline Twist

"I believe it is essential to be conscious of the total body. That is why I recommend a *twist* and *stretch* for this spot instead of a reach to the side."—Ron Fletcher

1. *Standing straight, body aligned, keep feet apart and facing straight ahead.*
2. *Raise your arms over your head, clasp your hands* (making sure that your hips continue to face forward).
3. *Twist.* Lift your body up—twist and bend down, touching your toes. If you can't touch them in the beginning, don't let that stop you. Keep doing this exercise and eventually you will find yourself reaching new lows.
4. *Touch your toes, come up.*
5. *Repeat on the other side.* Begin with three to each side and add three more each week until you are up to twelve on each side.

MAINTENANCE

21

MAINTENANCE

Maintenance is the biggest challenge of all. The thrill of watching the scale go down is over. The thrill of your new well-proportioned body makes you want to celebrate! So watch out. *You are reformed, not cured.*
A sugar addict—I am one—is reformed but never cured. Even now I know that I cannot control my intake of sugar. I know that if I had a bite of cake here and a spoonful of chocolate mousse there I'd be back into sugar full time. And I like the way I look now far too much to compromise. A moment's pleasure will never be worth losing my perfectly balanced figure.

The same thing is true of the fat addict. If you know that you can control yourself you can slowly add more foods containing fat or sugar. But always remember, you are reformed, never cured. If you go back to your old eating habits you will go back to your old lumpy, bumpy shape.

In my experience, when a person starts to act cured he goes hogwild. Bill illustrates this point perfectly. When he first came to me he was big all over but his stomach was huge from drinking too much beer. He lost 40 pounds over a four-month period. He looked great and felt great. At 55, after hitting the spot he had the body of a 30-year-old man. He exercised in conjunction with balancing his nutrients.

He was ready for Maintenance. He came in and said, "Hermien,

I will never get fat again! You don't have to warn me. I'm one of your clients you'll never have to worry about!"

Famous last words. That was Tuesday. Thursday Bill called and boasted, "I had a hot fudge sundae yesterday and my weight hasn't gone up an ounce. I told you nothing was gonna happen!"

Saturday he went to a wedding and Sunday to a christening. He had everything from champagne to wedding cake. Monday he called and said, "Guess what, Hermien? I haven't gained an ounce!"

I told him he was acting cured but it wasn't going to work. "One day—if not today, then tomorrow or the next day, or even the day after that—you're going to see a big jump in the scale."

"No, Hermien, not me. I'm not going overboard. Really."

Sure, I thought. Just wait . . .

Early Wednesday morning the phone rang. Bill asked if he could come and weigh himself. I asked him why. He said, "I think my scale's broken."

"What do you mean?" I asked him. "It was working all right Monday."

"Well, there's something wrong with it. I'm up ten pounds today. I'm ten pounds heavier than I was yesterday."

I told him to come in and weigh. He finally had to face reality. Sometimes it takes a few days before it shows. In his case the drinking showed in his face and his stomach. His spots were reappearing.

There is only one way to keep yourself in perfect shape and this is it:

Keeping in Perfect Shape

1. To begin Maintenance you should weigh three pounds less than your goal weight. This will allow your body to stabilize while increasing your intake of food. I would start with an extra ounce of protein or an extra piece of fruit. If you were fat from the waist down, start by increasing your carbohydrate intake, with, say, an extra piece of fruit or an extra piece of bread. You can add a *little* wine, but be cautious. Wine can awaken your sugar addiction and it can also make you relax your guard and lose control.
2. Weigh yourself every morning in the nude.
3. Take the following measurements once each week. Katharine Ross shows you how in the photo insert section of this book.

A. ARM MEASUREMENT
Place the end of the tape on your elbow and measure up until you've reached the largest part of your arm. Measure the circumference. Make sure that you always measure from the same point and the same distance up your arm.

B. CHEST MEASUREMENT
Wrap the tape around your back and measure the circumference. Use your nipples as a guideline. This goes for both men and women.

C. DIAPHRAGM MEASUREMENT
Measure from the center of your clavicle to the center of your diaphragm. Do it standing up and in front of a mirror.

D. WAISTLINE MEASUREMENT
Measure from the top of the hip bone to the smallest part of the waist.

E. ABDOMEN MEASUREMENT
Measure from the top of the hip bone to the biggest part of the abdomen.

F. POSTERIOR MEASUREMENT
Measure from the top of the hip bone to the biggest part of the behind.

G. THIGH MEASUREMENT
Measure up from the knee cap to the largest part of the thigh and take the circumference. Measure both thighs.

Always do them on the same day of the week, when you get up and in the nude. Remember: you can weigh the same and have two shapes. My clients who don't do this may stay at the same weight but their bodies will change—their spots will reappear or they will develop new ones.

4. If you go up a quarter of an inch on any one of those spots, go back on the program and it won't take you long to reduce. Do it immediately.

5. The longer you stay at a certain weight the more you will be able to eat or drink without gaining. You can never eat tremendous amounts but you *can eat anything* you can control. In my own case, I cannot control my intake of sugar. If I ate one cookie I would find it hard not to eat the whole box. Therefore, I eat cookies only once a year—on my birthday, when I give myself permission to lose control.

6. It usually takes two days for a weight gain to show up on the scale. Sometimes you'll eat something with salt in it and you may be retaining water, so don't panic. Don't use it as an excuse, either.
   When you weigh three pounds more than your goal weight for more than two days, go back on the base program until you have lost those three pounds.
7. You will be frightened at first, but experiment. If you find yourself losing control—if you have a sudden attack of hand-to-mouth disease or you just *have* to have another drink—stop! Toss whatever it is out! If you're in a restaurant, have it taken away immediately.
8. *Continue to play chess with food.* The more fattening the food, the less of it you may eat. Add more food *slowly*. And if you're going out to dinner and you know the food is going to be rich, leave off your bread and butter that day. If you have a very rich meal unexpectedly, leave off your bread and butter the following day. If you are confronted with something especially fattening, such as salmon mousse, pâté, or quiche, take small bites and don't finish the whole portion. Use good food sense. The longer you stabilize your weight the more you will be able to eat and drink.
9. Never leave out or refuse nutritious food in order to have something with empty calories. You will go into hidden hunger.
10. Follow the balance of protein, fat, and carbohydrate you learned while on the Master Plan. Add anything you can control. Continue taking a daily multivitamin/mineral. And remember: never have a carbohydrate without a protein unless you're going to bed.

Now that you know what caused your spots, it should be easier to keep them off in the future. Suzanne Somers has been one of my most successful clients. She and her husband, Alan Hamel, came to me nearly ten years ago. They both hit their spots and have maintained their well balanced bodies on a permanent basis.

One way Suzanne has been able to stay perfectly proportioned is by translating food into spots before she eats it. "Every once in a while," she says, "I have an ice cream sundae or a chocolate mousse and I think, 'Well, it's going right to my hips. It's going to take three weeks to get rid of it. Do I want it enough to eat it?' I know it's like taking the ice cream and slapping it on my legs where I used to have saddlebags. If I really want it I can have it now because I know how to counteract it and that I'm in control. I'll be thin when I'm ninety because I know how to maintain my weight and my shape."

Abigail Van Buren, known to millions of Americans as Dear Abby, came to me to trim her hips. She discovered that if she wanted to trim that spot she'd have to limit her intake of fried foods, cheese, and crisp chicken skin. "I learned a lot about nutrition," she says. "I learned food sense so that I can make wise decisions, especially when I'm out socially." Abby learned to play chess with food. She learned that eating fat-rich cheeses would make the spots on her hips reappear. "I used to love French Brie and Roquefort cheese," she explains, "and now I eat only the Laughing Cow Green label. As a result of being on the Spot Reducing Diet I'm able to maintain my weight."

When you go on Maintenance you have to be in control if you are going to be successful. I've had people come back to see me five years after they've hit their spots and still look as well proportioned and radiant as the day they walked out the door. They continued to follow the ten points outlined in this chapter and they were able to stay in control.

Dr. Joel Zisk, a Beverly Hills surgeon, lost 38 pounds on the program and has kept it off for over three years. "There are many fad diets," he says. "People go up and down like elevators. I was tired of that. I wanted to stabilize my weight once and for all. In my opinion, the best part of the Spot Reducing Diet is the Maintenance diet. Once you've lost the weight you can keep it off! And believe me, that's the real plus!"

Always remember: It takes only 50 extra calories per meal, or 150 extra calories a day, to make you 15 pounds heavier in one year!

Maintenance Measurements

	INCHES	DATE	DATE	DATE
1. ARMS				
2. BUST				
3. DIAPHRAGM				
4. WAIST				
5. STOMACH				
6. POSTERIOR				
7. THIGHS				

APPENDIX A

Questions and Answers

After working with more than 4000 people, I've discovered that there are number of questions I'm asked repeatedly. I've included them because I think that they may help you hit the spot.

1. Do I need vitamins when I diet?

    To insure an adequate diet, note the recommended daily allowances based on a 2000-calorie-a-day diet put out by the Food and Nutrition Board, National Academy of Sciences, National Research Council. Since you'd have to be almost a giant to lose weight eating that many calories a day, a vitamin supplement allows you to eat fewer calories (or less food) while still getting your essential nutrients.

2. What if I don't eat but take vitamins, minerals, and protein powders?

    When you rely on pills and powders, you're not getting the full range of nutrients. There is so much in nutrition that has yet to be discovered. In a variety of food, one will not only receive the known nutrients, but also those yet to be discovered. Pills and powders provide only *some* of the things you need.

3. Will a diet soda and a bowl of iceberg lettuce help me reduce faster?

    Yes, it certainly will. You'll reduce your looks, your health, and your weight.

4. Does toasting cut down calories?
   No, it does not.

5. Does eating at bedtime make you gain weight faster?
   Calories do not increase in value just because you go to bed. Your body works all night anyway and you may weigh more in the morning because of salt and water content. Your weight is based on your intake and exercise in a 24-hour period. Your digestive system works when you're asleep as well as when you're awake.

6. I eat almost nothing, but I can't seem to lose weight. Why is that?
   Eating small quantities of food can add up to a large calorie count. Fifty extra calories a meal or 150 extra calories a day will add up to 15 extra pounds in a year. It is universally accepted that you must burn more calories than you consume in order to lose weight.

7. May I add salt to boiling water for cooking vegetables?
   Much of what we eat contains high amounts of salt. We do not need to add any more. Too much salt can contribute to hypertension. *Do not use it.* Instead of salt, use any spice or herb you like but never anything like garlic salt or onion salt.

8. Don't we need salt?
   Yes, but you get enough from natural foods and restaurant foods, over which we have no control.

9. Is honey better than sugar?
   Honey has a little more riboflavin and potassium than sugar but it doesn't carry enough vitamins and minerals to make it worth risking sugar addiction.

10. Can I eat too much fruit?
    Fruit is good only as it provides vitamins and minerals for the body. Too much becomes excess sugar and will cause you to gain weight and enhance your spots from the waist up.

11. Why isn't it all right just to have a green salad for lunch?
    Salads are made up of carbohydrates. Carbohydrates leave the stomach quickly, get into the bloodstream, give you a rush of energy, then let you down. When you have a protein, such as a hard-boiled egg, in conjunction with carbohydrate, the protein breaks down at a slower rate, thus keeping you from having a low-mood swing by giving you continuous energy.

12. What's wrong with dieting all week and just bingeing on the weekend?

    Bingeing is what puts lumps and bumps on your shape. One piece of candy a day is better than seven on Saturday, though *none* is best of all. It's easier when a person can learn not to want it. If you can't control it, you can't have it. That goes for any food.

13. Is there any food that isn't fattening?

    Any food can be fattening if you eat too much of it.

14. Is it good to drink water with meals?

    As long as water doesn't replace the foods you need for good nutrition, it's fine. It's good to drink several glasses of water a day.

15. Won't I always have some cravings?

    The longer a person's away from something, the less he or she thinks about it. The things you love you may always crave, but the cravings will be fewer and further apart.

16. Will I gain faster by eating junk food than other food?

    Junk food can contain vitamins, minerals, and protein but it also contains a lot of fat and sugar and salt, which make it high in calories. For example, a big, greasy fast-food cheeseburger with mayonnaise and ketchup, plus a bag of French fries, plus two other medium-sized meals during the day will make a person gain weight.

17. How is the Spot Reducing Diet different from the Weight Watchers regime?

    The Spot Reducing Diet is less regimented than the program of Weight Watchers. One can eat as little as two or as many as six meals a day. As one of my clients says, "I prefer the Spot Reducing Diet because it allows me to be so flexible. When I was on Weight Watchers, I was always frightened of eating away from home."

18. If I'm well fed, won't I be well nourished?

    No, not necessarily. One can be well fed on junk foods without being well nourished. "Well nourished" means that you're getting the nutrients that make your body work well as opposed to foods with empty calories such as cookies that do nothing but taste good. They may give you a quick, short-lived burst of energy but they will give you big, ugly spots.

19. Are all additives and preservatives bad for you?
    No; in fact some additives and preservatives are necessary to fight harmful bacteria—but use fresh food when possible.

20. Is it O.K. to cook with wine?
    Yes, because the alcohol burns off, getting rid of many of the calories.

21. I get so bloated and retain water. Why?
    Either from eating too much salt, MSG, or too much carbohydrate for the amount of protein and fat that you eat.

22. Is exercise important?
    Physical activity is an essential element in appetite and weight control. It is actually an appetite deterrent.

23. Why can I have only one ounce of cheese a day?
    Cheese is a nutritious food but it is not only high in cholesterol, it is also high in fat. Too much will enhance your spots from the waist down.

24. Why is it O.K. to eat baked potatoes but not mashed potatoes?
    A plain baked potato is not fattening—it's the company it keeps. Mashed potatoes usually have cream or milk and butter and salt added. If you add nothing, you can have mashed potatoes. Hidden ingredients make your spots bigger.

25. Should I stay away from red meat?
    Everything is all right in moderation. Once or twice a week is fine but don't have highly marbled meat; the white part is fat. The less expensive cuts, such as flank steak, are usually less fatted than Porterhouse.

26. I love gelatin desserts. Are they O.K. to eat?
    No. They are empty calories. You do not need sugar.

27. I want to stop smoking but I'm afraid I will gain weight. What can I do?
    You will gain weight if you replace cigarettes with food. Eat low-calorie foods while you're going through nicotine withdrawal.

28. What's wrong with just counting calories?

First, one can have apple pie and cheese and be within a certain caloric limit, thus being well fed but not well nourished. Second, calorie charts differ so much. There are many reasons: size of portion, preparation, and degree of fat. Amounts are also often hard to pin down, such as food amounts measured in inches.

APPENDIX B

ABOUT YOUR BODY

PROTEIN

Proteins form the basis of all living organisms. The structure of every living cell is formed by protein. Therefore protein is essential to forming life as well as sustaining it.

Every day, millions of cells break down and protein rebuilds them. Protein is tied up with the immune system, so if you become protein-deficient your immune system will break down and leave you open to all kinds of disease. We've all allowed ourselves to work too hard, play too hard, or become exhausted and forget to eat properly; when that happens the body lets us know by getting a cold or the flu.

Part of protein's job is to act as transport for enzymes and hormones. We each have over 4000 enzymes and numerous hormones. They must be nourished, and protein, in my opinion, is essential to their proper nourishment. When they are properly nourished they give the body wonderful service.

When they become deprived and undernourished they don't seem to function very well. I've worked with women in their sixties who have gone from deprivation to reward all their lives and no matter what they do, they can't lose weight. They have followed my program and after losing only a few pounds they reach a plateau and stay there. I'm convinced that their enzymes and hormones have been thrown off balance. My solution is to send those clients to an endocrinologist for testing.

Protein has the ability to break down into carbohydrate when necessary. It is also involved with the genetic code. Depending on how pure the protein is, it can stimulate metabolism as much as 30 percent. Carbohydrate stimulates metabolism only 6 percent. But remember, if you consume too much protein you will also be getting fat.

Learn which foods are included in the protein category. This information will help you develop good food sense.

Complete Proteins

Complete proteins are those that contain all eight essential amino acids. Scientists are still debating the ninth. The body neither makes nor stores these amino acids so you must get them from your daily diet. These proteins are of animal origin.

- meat
- fish
- poultry
- milk
- eggs
- cheese

Soybeans are the most complete of the vegetable proteins, though they lack some methionine.

Incomplete Proteins

Incomplete proteins are those deficient in one or more of the essential amino acids. They are of plant origin.

- grains
- legumes
- nuts

In a well-balanced diet, animal and plant proteins work to supplement one another. Vegetarians must be careful to get the necessary amount of protein, especially when they eat little or no protein.

Protein Exchange

A few examples of how you can substitute one protein for another:

SUBSTITUTE	FOR
nonfat milk	whole milk or lowfat
tuna or chicken in water	tuna or chicken in oil
lobster with lemon juice	lobster with melted butter
oysters on half shell	oyster stew
chicken	duck
chicken breasts	chicken legs

Carbohydrate Exchange

Here are a few examples of how you can substitute one carbohydrate for another. Select a carbohydrate that is low in calories instead of one that is *loaded*.

SUBSTITUTE	FOR
baked potato, 2½" diameter	mashed potatoes (1 cup)
puffed rice (1 cup)	granola (1 cup)
1 cup green beans	1 cup baked beans
1 cup asparagus	1 cup lima beans
diet soft drink	regular soft drink
tomato juice	bloody Mary
sponge cake—2" slice	iced chocolate cake

Carbohydrates are classified in three primary groups:

MONOSACCHARIDES—simple sugars that cannot be broken down into smaller units. Glucose, fructose, and galactose.

fruits	fruit juice
vegetables	tonic water
hard candy	honey
soft drinks	

DISACCHARIDES—more nearly complete sugars; sucrose, maltose, and lactose

table sugar
brown sugar
molasses
syrup

milk (lactose is the sugar)
malt
ketchup

POLYSACCHARIDES—complex molecules made up of many sugars combined, starch and cellulose

potatoes
rice
cereal and cereal grains
legumes
corn starch

flour
pasta, noodles, macaroni
bread and rolls
seeds